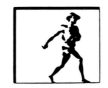

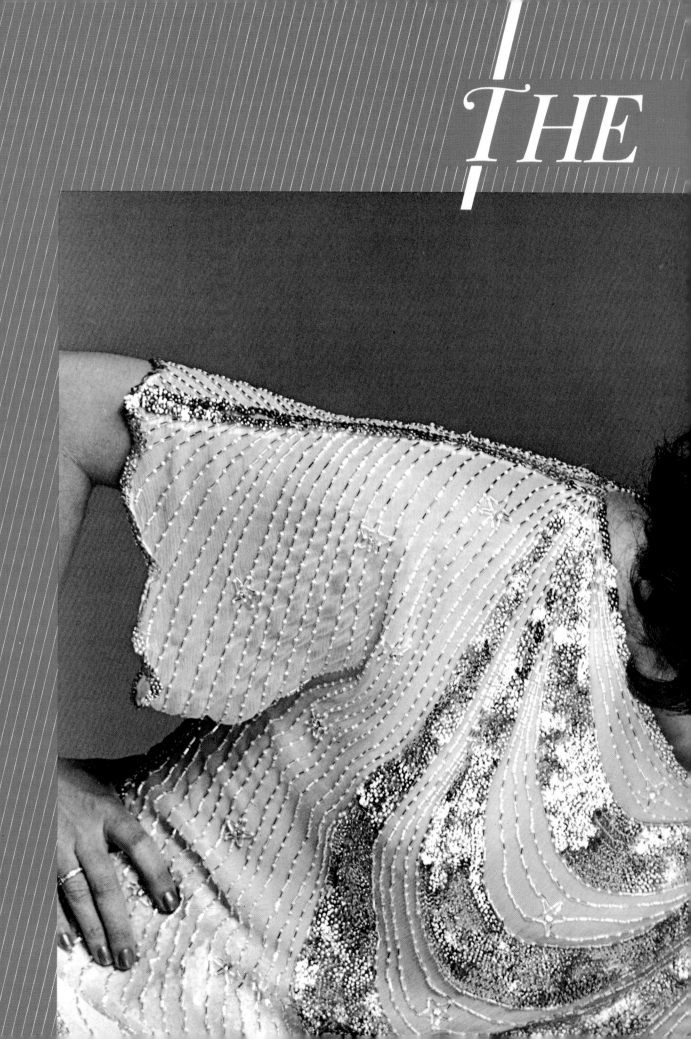

THE

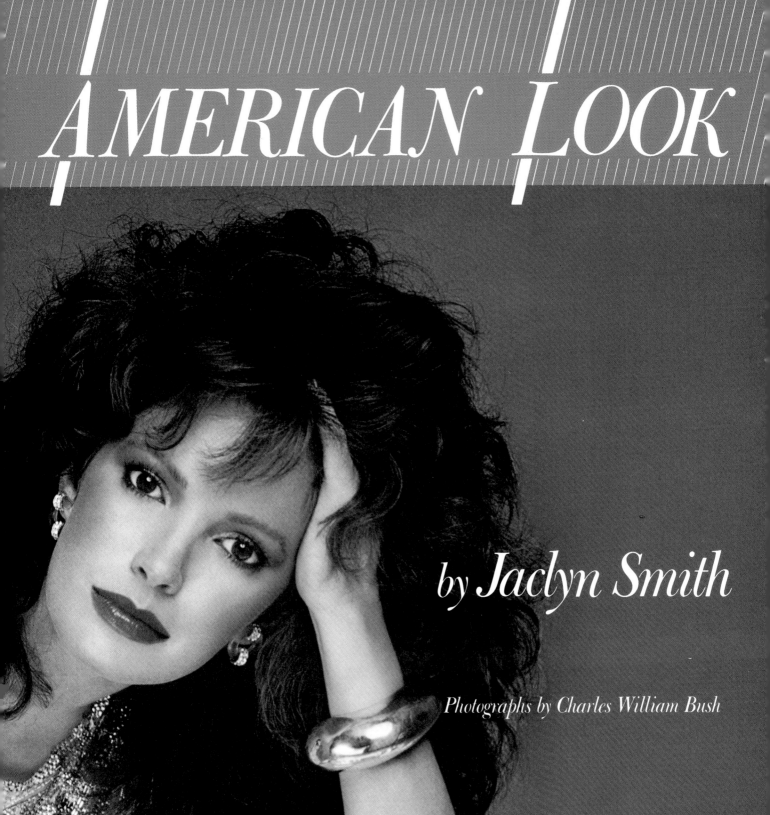

AMERICAN LOOK

by *Jaclyn Smith*

Photographs by Charles William Bush

SIMON AND SCHUSTER
New York

Text copyright © 1984 by Jaclyn Smith
Photographs copyright © 1984 by Charles William Bush

Published by Simon and Schuster
A Division of Simon & Schuster, Inc.
Simon & Schuster Building
Rockefeller Center
1230 Avenue of the Americas
New York, New York 10020

SIMON AND SCHUSTER and colophon are registered trademarks of Simon & Schuster, Inc.

Designed by Levavi & Levavi

Drawings by Lamont O'Neal

Production Directed by Richard L. Willett

Manufactured in the United States of America

10   9   8   7   6   5   4   3   2   1

Library of Congress Cataloging in Publication Data

Smith, Jaclyn.
  The American Look.

  1. Beauty, Personal. 2. Hairdressing. 3. Skin—Care
and hygiene. 4. Cosmetics. I. Title. II. Title: Beauty
book.
RA778.S63   1984   646.7'042   84-20296

ISBN: 0-671-50172-0

For Margaret Ellen Smith,
the most beautiful woman I know,
who more importantly happens to be my mother

And for my son, Gaston Anthony Richmond,
who on March 19, 1982,
made me the happiest woman in the whole world

Contents

THE
AMERICAN
LOOK

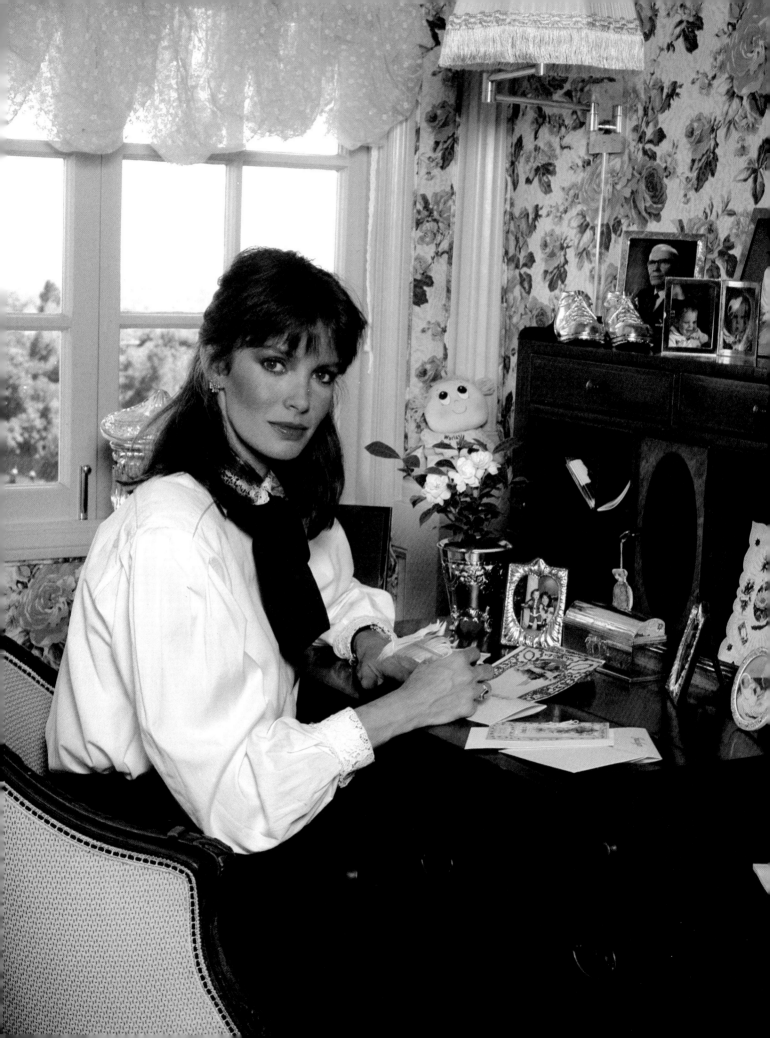

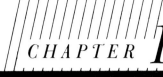

CHAPTER 1

Through the Years: My Mirror Image

You know, I might never have written a beauty book like this if it weren't for you. That's right. I hardly consider myself the world's ultimate expert in anything, including beauty. But because of the countless fabulous letters I've received and all the people who have come up to me on the street—with so many specific questions about diet, makeup, hair—I've finally done it.

As appreciative as I am of people's sincere interest in me, I've never really had enough time to answer all these important questions thoroughly. I've always tried to reply to your letters, but I wanted to do more in response to your appeals and enthusiasm. And so I decided to write down all my ideas about beauty in a book.

Although I'm flattered that many people believe that I typify "The American Look," I'm hardly the Wizard of Oz in the realm of beauty. But I have learned so much from the demands of my television, commercial, fashion and film work—and from the experts in those fields. I can't supply three magic tips that'll make you a movie star overnight, but I can share with you my carefully considered advice and pass on what seems to work for me.

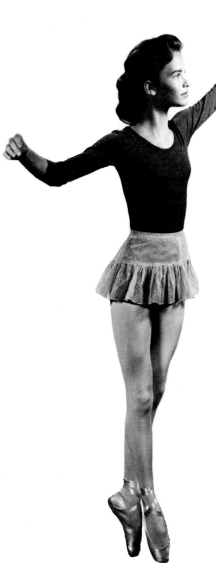

Ballet became an obsession when I was about eleven.

Believability, the essence of The American Look, has always been very important to me—as an actress, as a woman. And that attitude doesn't allow for tricked-up, faddish looks anytime—in front of the camera, at a gala opening, or at home with my husband and son. Any woman, actress or not, looks most attractive, most appealing, when she's made an effort to capitalize on whatever assets she may possess.

I suppose what I'm saying—and I know you've heard it before—is that you have to like you as *yourself,* not as your approximation of an image on a magazine cover or a face on a television screen. I did not write this book to turn out thousands of Jaclyn Smith look-alikes, but rather to inspire you, if I can, to become the prettiest *you* possible.

First, let me assure you that I didn't grow up constantly looking at myself in the mirror, assessing, nurturing, judging my looks from moment to moment. Whatever attractiveness I did have as a young schoolgirl wasn't much commented on. That just wasn't the way my family worked. I wasn't encouraged to be vain at all. Now I have to admit that I did win our school's "Most Beautiful" contest when I was in the seventh grade. But I also have to tell you that at that age, winning the sixty-yard dash was just as thrilling for me. And most thrilling of all was ballet.

Not unlike many little girls growing up in relatively comfortable circumstances in Houston, I was given ballet lessons. I began at about age three, but at that point it was simply the prettiness of ballet that delighted me. At about age eleven, I became obsessed with the skills involved, the relationship between music and the body's movement, and with the challenge of precision that ballet requires. And I really mean obsessed! I was always dancing. My mother really had to watch over me, otherwise, when we'd go shopping, I'd be doing grand jetés down the aisles. Even when I was standing still, I would stand in first or second position.

Looking back, I see that this fierce interest had its pros and cons. On the one hand, I received tremendous training as a dancer, and established attitudes of body awareness and fitness that stand me in good stead today. I also learned personal discipline. But on the other hand, my absorption with dance pulled me out of the mainstream of high school and college life. All the usual things, football games, school parties and cliques and cheerleading, took a backseat for me.

Not that I was a total loner. I did participate in things like school dramatics, but basically I lived, breathed and slept dance.

I know what you're thinking—that the age of discovery—*boys*—must have had an impact on me, especially on my attitude toward my looks. But it really didn't. I dated, of course. But always one boy at a time. I wasn't the kind who tried to attract the attention of lots of boys.

Maybe it sounds a little backward, but I never begged to wear that all-important first pair of high heels; I wasn't dying to get a chance to wear lipstick. In fact, my tastes ran to the other extreme; I truly preferred wearing sneakers and no makeup. Clean, clear skin and shining hair was my "look."

Perhaps surprisingly, my look and attitude didn't change much after I came to New York to study acting and find work as a dancer. I think my parents' love and support played a big role in enabling me to be so much my own person, so little swayed by my peers. I grew up knowing I was loved and that they were proud of me, as a person, even before I had any notable accomplishments to my credit. They also understood my decision to leave college after only one year to pursue my real interests. I only hope that I can offer that rare kind of uncritical support to my own son, Gaston.

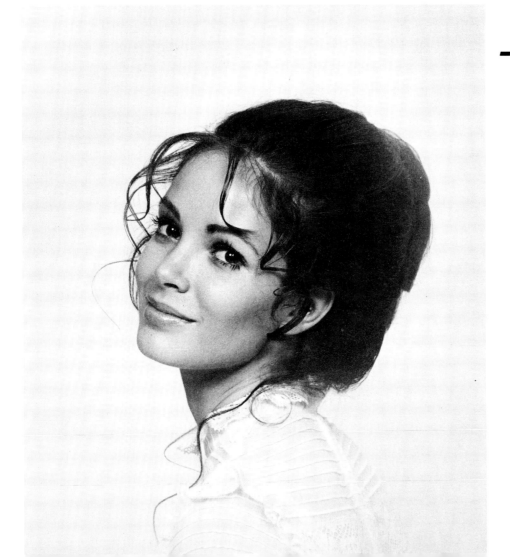

From my portfolio, my first year modeling in New York City

*From my modeling
portfolio a year later, with
the long straight hair so
popular in the late sixties*

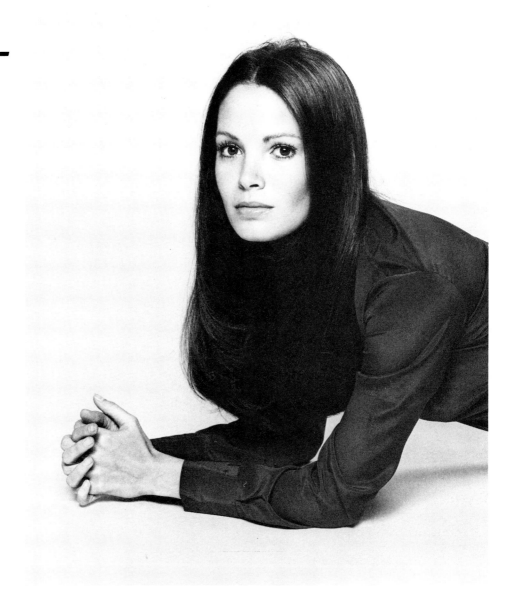

I considered those first exciting years in New York more valuable than another three of college. I received excellent training, matured and sorted out my goals. For one thing, I discovered that the total dedication to the art and craft demanded of the professional ballerina was not for me. I was too much of a homebody and definitely wanted a family someday. So—shades of the movie *The Turning Point*—I vaguely planned to return to Houston one day to open a ballet school. I loved the idea of teaching dance.

Fate, however, had different plans. I had been accepted for a touring, summer-stock production of *Gypsy* when a polyp on my vocal cords forced me to drop out of rehearsal. It was heartbreaking, because I'd found musical comedy a very enticing alternative to ballet. The whole idea of Broadway was fascinating.

About the same time, I was one of several people who responded to a notice posted backstage calling for people who thought they could do commercials. I went to see the agency, and suddenly, I found myself signed up and sent off to shoot a Listerine commercial. There was the usual hiatus till my next job, for Camay soap, but then things really began to click. It was a whole new world to me and a wonderful way to make a living. I was quite intrigued and challenged with learning how to look and act on film and how to get a message across in only thirty seconds.

It was from a commercial that I got my first television-series acting assignment, on "McCloud," and continued success in series appearances led me to move to Hollywood, and, after a couple of years, to "Charlie's Angels." That show was a tremendous success. But as my career took this totally unexpected path, I was able to maintain my

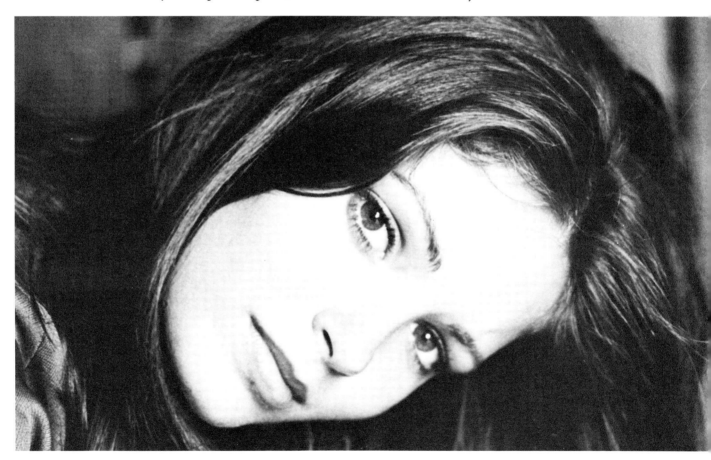

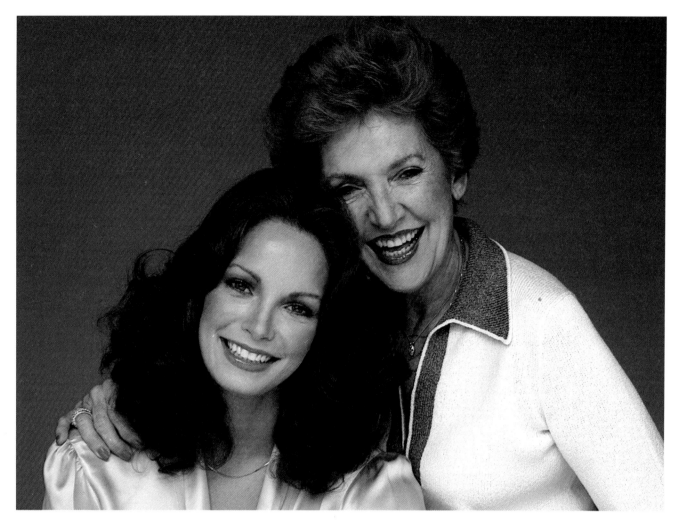

With my mother, Margaret Ellen Smith, who taught me that being happy is the true essence of beauty

balance because of the strong, simple values I was brought up with— my belief in honesty, hard work, and the family.

People often ask about the competition and insecurity that so frequently plague women in my profession, but I had never been seriously threatened by those traps. I think the reason was partly because, not being a true fashion model, I didn't have the obsession that my look was the only thing I had to offer. I had very real dancing, and then acting, skills to back me up. And, fortunately, I was never that desperate about wanting a career. Even today, when I'm busier and working harder than ever before, my family life comes first.

I don't mean to sound like a Pollyanna. Certainly I had disappointments, roles I wanted that I didn't get. And there were times when I'd say to myself, "Gee, if only my legs weren't so like a dancer's, maybe if they were a little fuller at the thigh . . ." But I never wanted

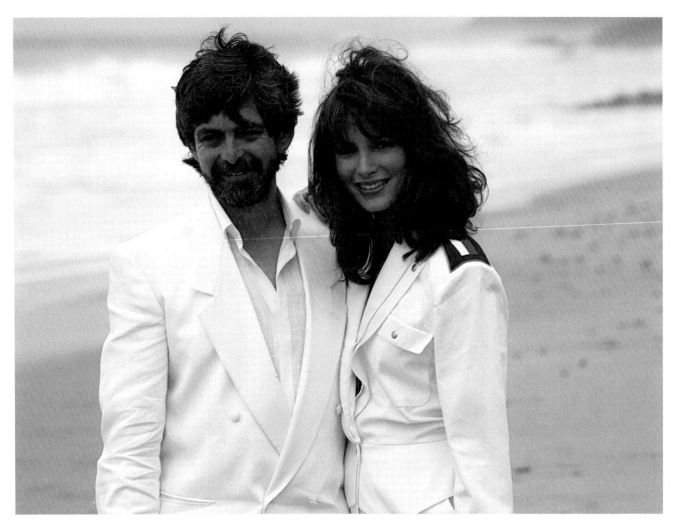

to look like anyone else, or be anyone else. Nor did I ever seriously consider dramatically changing my look. I was bolstered by my hard-earned talent and my family's supportive attitude to say, "If they want me, fine: If they don't want me, that's okay, too. But if they want me to be somebody else, well, that just doesn't make any sense at all."

If I did hit a stretch where I was getting a little confused or frenetic about my career, I would call on my parents. To this day, when I'm feeling pressured or troubled and need just a dash of realism, or perspective, they're there, with wise, loving counsel. And believe me, things can get pretty tangled and crazy being married to Tony Richmond, an Academy Award–winning cinematographer who's often my producer or director as well. Since my parents are not involved in the business, they can always offer the proverbial "breath of fresh air."

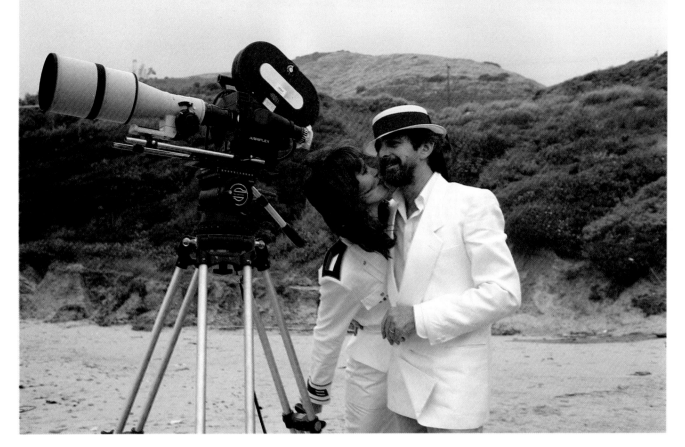

All this mom-and-apple-pie stuff might sound a bit strange coming from a thrice-married actress. But even though my first two marriages didn't work out—the first time I was too young; the second was a question of competition and conflicting schedules between two actors trying to live together—I still believe that each marriage was initially based on the right stuff.

Deciding whether a man's interest in me was genuine has never been a big problem for me. I trust my intuition. Plus, my life-style has always served as a sort of natural selection process. I'm a definite, even opinionated person, and my life-style is not Hollywood's. I may live in the heart of Bel Air, but I'm not into drugs; I'm not into wild partying or going night after night to restaurants to see and be seen. Any man looking for that kind of life with Jaclyn Smith would be, quite simply, out of luck.

In truth, I'm a romantic who clings to heart and hearth. I'm a woman who delights in feminine things—lace, hearts and flowers—and looking pretty for the two men in my life, and for myself.

If I had become that housewife/dance teacher, living down the street from my parents in Houston, I'd surely be a lot less concerned with my looks. But it would be disingenuous of me to say that my chosen career doesn't place demands on me for careful and consistent attention to beauty. After all, I see daily rushes when I'm shooting a film; I see the advertisements and magazine covers I've posed for. I've arrived at some very definite ideas about how I look, and what I like. But, like anyone else, I also have a husband whom I love and for whom I want to be attractive. And I notice the little things that change with age and experience.

Beauty is, of course, big business for a lot of people. But let me pause a moment to express my sincere feelings about overindulgence in this whole topic. Particularly in my profession, one meets or comes across people who are solely focused on their physical appearance. And I'm quite certain that that sort of tunnel vision makes them less attractive, because it makes them less happy people.

A healthy sense of balance and acceptance is the key. For instance, since Gaston's birth about two years ago, I've noticed a slightly dark patch on one cheekbone that requires a little special attention in terms of studio makeup. I've also noticed that my face is a bit thinner now than before his birth, giving me wonderfully pronounced cheekbones,

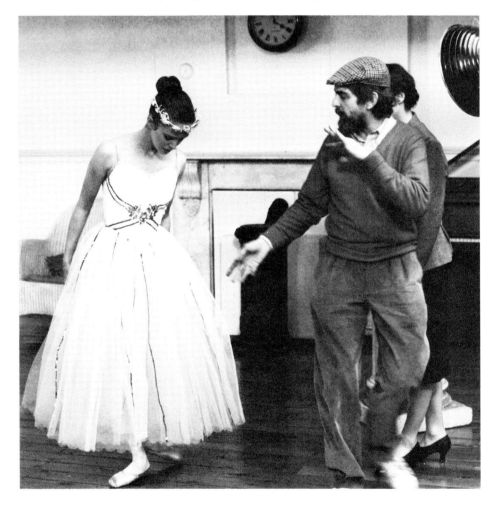

Tony directing me in a scene from the movie **Déjà Vu**

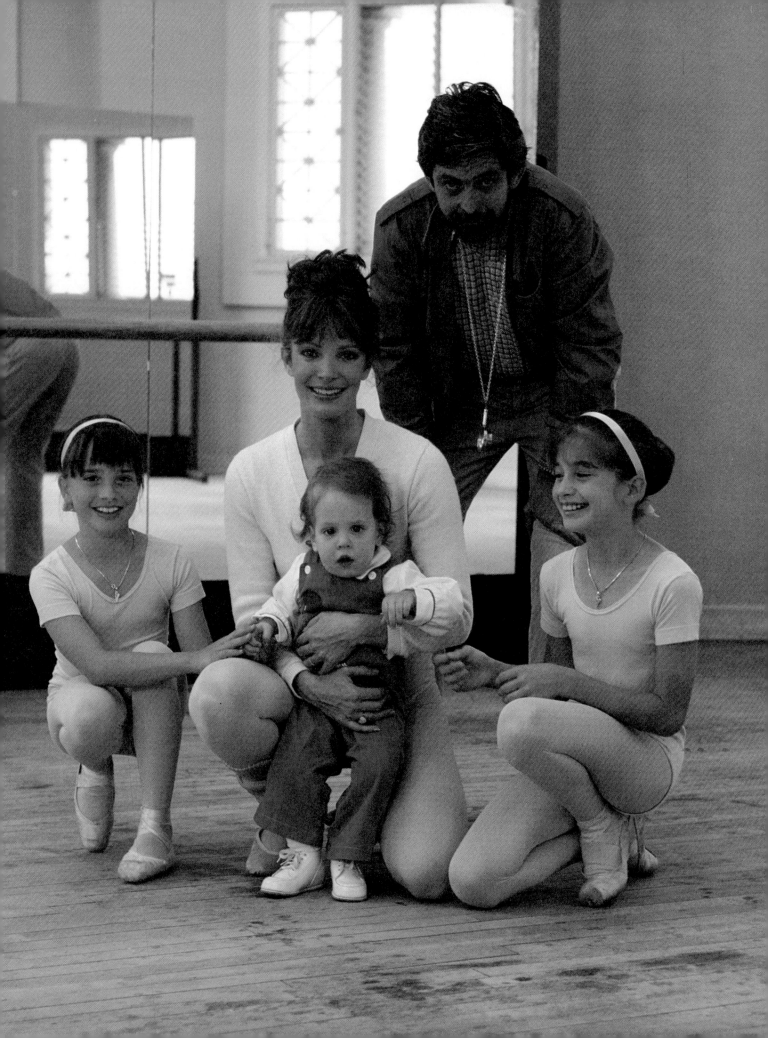

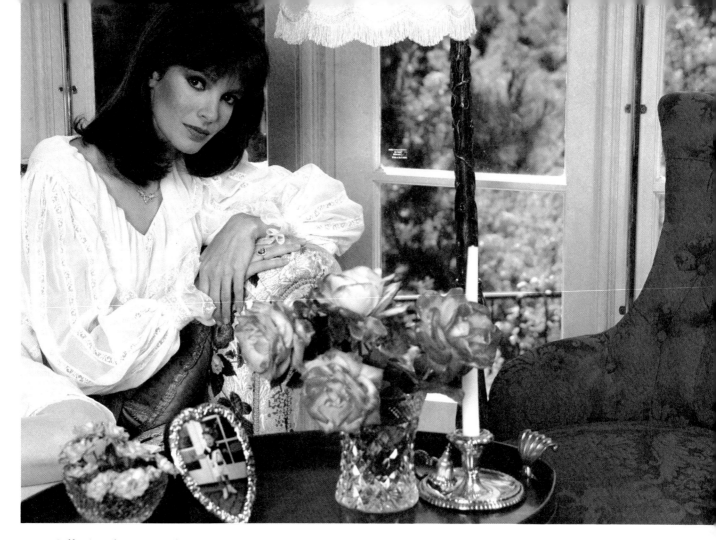

especially in photographs. So you see—you lose some, you win some!

I'm proud to typify The American Look, grateful to be considered a beautiful woman, and I'm adamant about taking care of my looks. But I'm not going to become a slave to them, either.

I suspect that part of my down-to-earth, straightforward attitude toward beauty has to do with having a mother who was and is fantastic looking, yet who would never dream of torturing herself over her looks. How much of that self-assurance she would attribute to good, clean living and years with a man who adores her and thinks she's the most beautiful woman on earth, I don't know. But she sets a great example.

I can't promise you an adoring man, or, as I said, a movie career. But we can certainly work together on a great new look for you.

(opposite): Tony and Gaston visiting me on the set of a commercial shoot for Max Factor. With us are Elkin and Angelique Antonio, daughters of old family friend Lou Antonio.

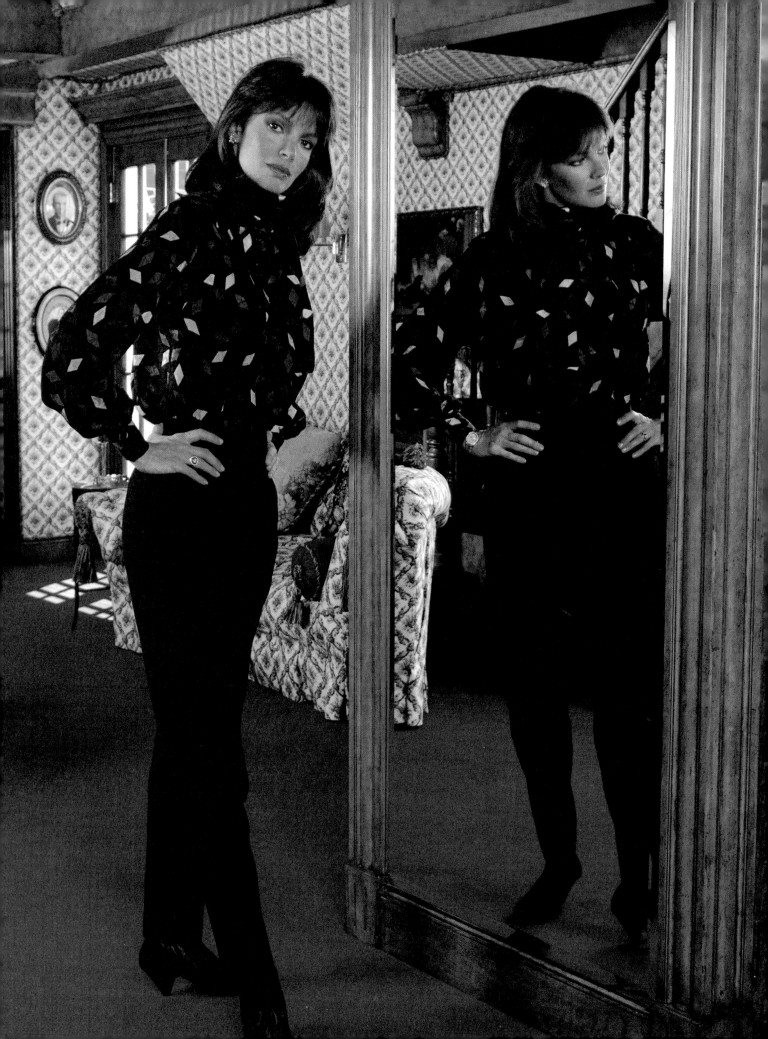

CHAPTER 2

Take a Good, Long Look

We've talked about me, now let's talk about you and your beauty goals. In general, we've agreed that you want to look, and feel, as good as possible, right? That calls for a head-to-toe self-analysis.

To start, stand about ten to fifteen feet in front of a full-length mirror, dressed, coiffed and made up as you would be on a normal day. Look at yourself as if you were passing yourself on the street, and try to get the fresh, unbiased view of a casual passerby. (This isn't as ridiculous as it seems. After all, at least half the reason we even bother to make the most of our appearance is for other people, isn't it?)

What are the first three things you notice? Don't hesitate; don't think about whether they are positive or negative. Just react as spontaneously and objectively as possible. (This is almost like an improvisational acting-class assignment.)

Now jot down those first three "noticeables" and evaluate them. If you've written, for instance, "hair," does it mean your hairstyle is overpowering or your color too brassy, or that your hair is shiny and beautiful, a real standout beauty asset? If you've written down "hips," it's probably not one for the positive column. But try to analyze whether you notice your hips because you're truly too hippy, or because the skirt or pants you've chosen, in combination with your blouse or sweater, misemphasizes an otherwise proportional figure. If you've noted "mouth," it may be that your lipstick shade is too strong, overwhelming the other features of your face, or that it's appealing, even luscious—a real quality to be played up. You get the idea.

I believe this kind of self-analysis is a way to pick out some realistic beauty pluses as well as points of potential improvement. Directly asking others' opinions can be dangerous. At best, it can lead to confusion; at worst, hurt feelings. Trust your own objective impressions.

YOUR BODY

For the next step in your head-to-toe self-analysis, take off your clothes, and again, standing far enough away from the mirror to get a full-length view, check out your body's proportions, front and back. Your eye will tell you what needs improvement: waist too full, bottom too big, thighs too pudgy, whatever.

The bare facts of problem areas are right in front of you. And improvements can be made with consistent spot exercise or a diet-plus-exercise plan that takes into account your metabolism, your number of fat cells and your overall muscle tone. But first, it's important to set *realistic* standards and goals for yourself.

In this age of science and technology, many of us have become fascinated with measuring ourselves. Although such methods applied to body type are only partially useful because of wide variations in human body configurations due to heredity and other factors, get out your measuring tape and scales, if you like. We'll run through some commonly used quantifiers.

As a general rule of thumb, you can check your weight against this equation: a woman five feet tall = 100 pounds. For every inch over five feet, add another 3 pounds to determine your ideal weight. At five feet seven inches, I am allowed 121 pounds, except that we haven't yet taken my on-the-small-side frame into consideration. Ultimately, I should subtract a few pounds for being small-boned to reach an ideal of approximately 117 pounds. (That's actually 2 pounds over my personal ideal weight.) Even so, this formula yields a lower

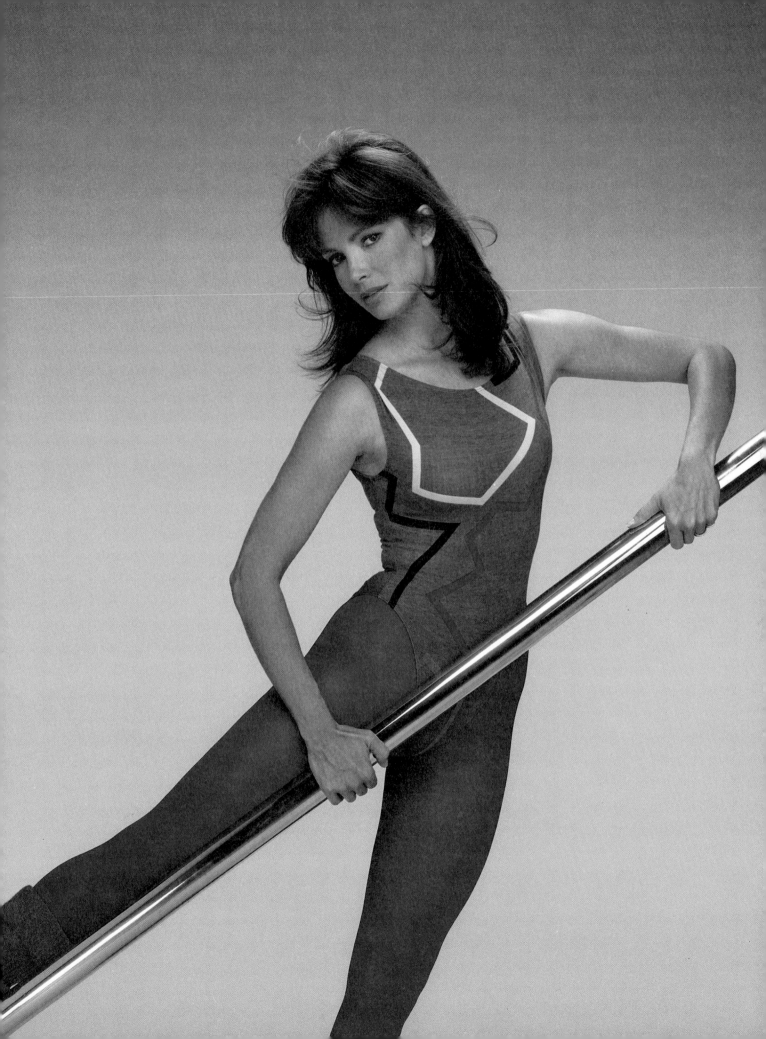

figure than those found on often-cited insurance-company charts, and is more realistic if you're after a more "fashionable" body. If you're big-boned, you should add a few pounds.

If you don't know whether you're big- medium- or small-framed, whip out your measuring tape and follow me. Measure your wrist just above the protruding bone. If it's less than 5½ inches, it's small; if it's between 5½ and 6½ inches, it's medium, and over 6½ inches is considered big.

A third measurement you can try is the pelvic bone. Measure across your tummy, from protruding point to protruding point. (Yes, you can, in fact, should, suck in your stomach.) If the width is 8 inches or less, it's small; 8 to 10 inches is medium and over 10 inches, large.

Since every body is so individually shaped, all three of these measurements need not fall into the same category. Two undoubtedly will, and the three considered together can give you a rough image of your skeletal shape and size. (Remember that your frame is not something you can alter.)

Now that you know your general body-frame size, you can go back and adjust your ideal weight. And depending how far off your current weight is, you may want to take a jog around the block, sign up for at least another twenty aerobics classes, or stop for a piece of chocolate cake.

But wait. Pounds aren't everything. It depends on what your scale is registering: pounds of fat, pounds of muscle, pounds of flesh. Thin women can be flabby, even have cellulite, if they have unworked or underdeveloped muscles. If you are in good shape, with ultratoned muscles, your actual weight could exceed the ideal for the simple reason that muscle is heavier than fat.

There are several ways to determine the percentage of body fat you're carrying around with you. The least scientific is the tried-and-true pinch test. Simply pinch the flesh at strategic locations—upper arms, hips, backs of thighs—and scold yourself if you can pinch more than an inch.

At health spas and sport-medicine clinics, experts will often use calipers to determine the percentage of body fat. (Tennis champion Martina Navratilova has said that reducing her percentage of body fat was a primary goal in her dramatic and admirable shape-up of several years ago.) Or, they'll do a submersion test. This rather damp and complicated procedure requires that you be weighed before your entire body is lowered into a tank full of water. You're weighed again submerged, and through calculations involving the known mass of

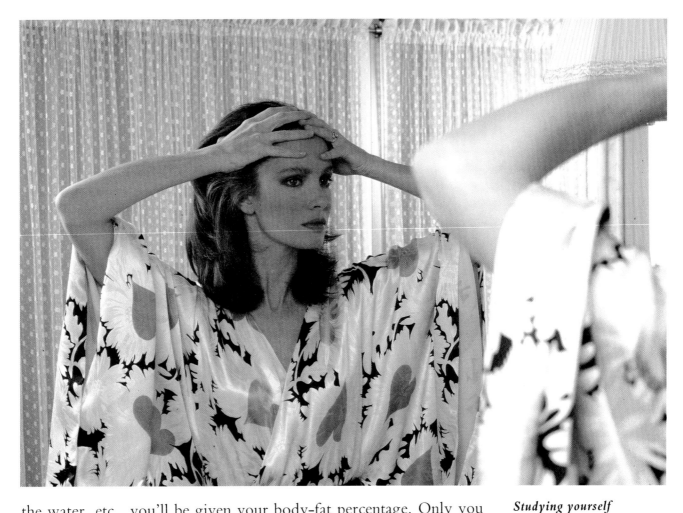

the water, etc., you'll be given your body-fat percentage. Only you can decide if that's worth the procedure.

Models often use a general principle of proportional measurements that you may also want to try. The idea is that your bust and hip measurements be within one or two inches of each other, and that your waist be, optimally, ten or twelve inches less than your bust.

Okay, now that you've arrived at a fairly realistic assessment of your body, you can get dressed again. But whether or not you've followed along with these statistical formulas, the fact remains that how you *feel* in your body—sluggish and embarrassed, or light and agile—is what really matters more than anything else. Besides, there are too many individual variables to arrive at the perfect body on paper. It'll be done in *your* exercise class; at the table as *you* sit down to eat; in the boutiques or stores as *you* buy your clothes—all of which we'll discuss in the chapters that follow.

Studying yourself carefully, even critically, yields your best hair and makeup looks.

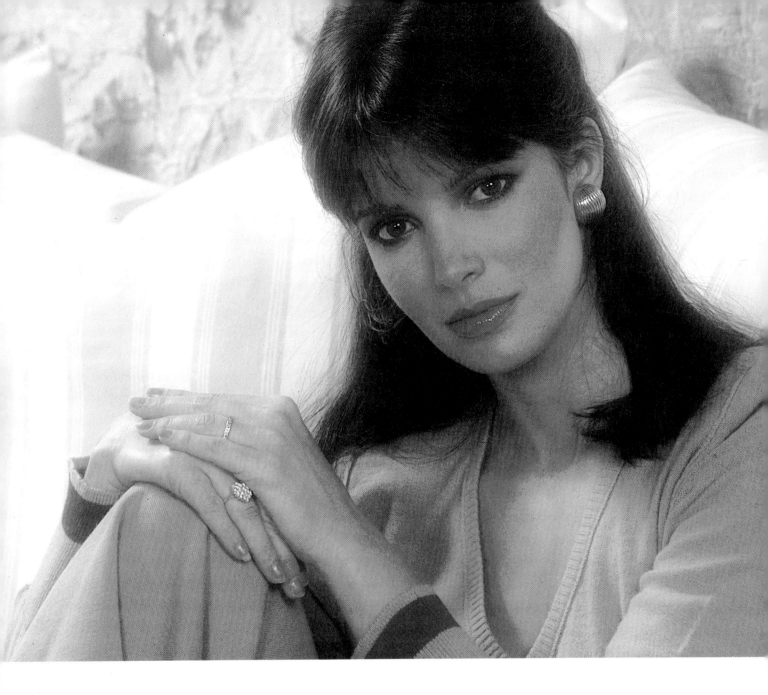

YOUR FACE AND HAIR

Now let's take a close look in a well-lighted mirror. At this range, try another "first-three" list of things that grab your attention. That practically invisible scar over your right eye? A chin that's less than strong? Compelling blue eyes? A too-wide nose? A sensuous mouth? An oily patch midforehead? These are precisely the points—the beauty assets and drawbacks—you'll want to keep in mind to enhance and diminish respectively, with appropriate skin care and makeup.

But if you find yourself gazing into the mirror and wishing you looked exactly like Rita Hayworth or Marilyn Monroe or your sister's best friend, forget it. You have to be sincerely happy with and interested in being *you* for anyone's beauty advice to be of value. (Think about it: where would Rita and Marilyn have gotten if *they* wanted to look like Greta Garbo?)

We live in an era that celebrates the individual—in terms of appearance and accomplishments—so let's take advantage of that. All you need is healthy self-interest when it comes to achieving your best complexion, your most flattering hairstyle and makeup, your best overall look.

Let's get started!

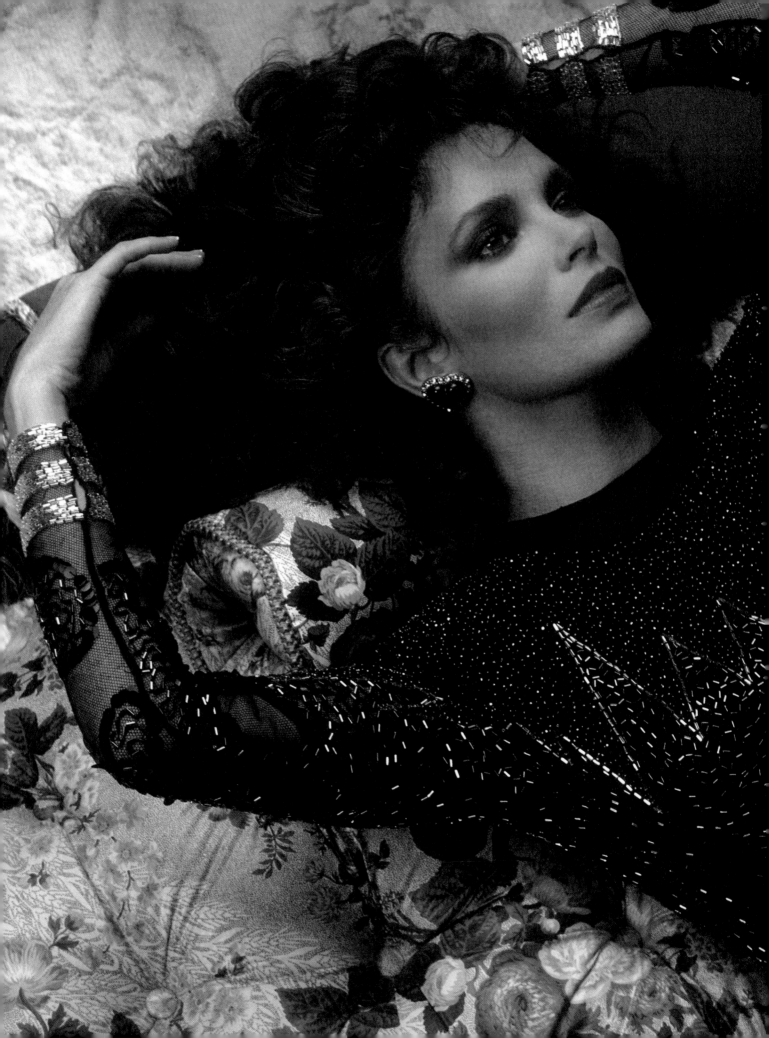

CHAPTER 3

Hair Today: Glorious Tomorrow

My hair has been a prominent feature of my professional image, which is fine because it's the one beauty- or fashion-related aspect of my appearance I've always been interested in. I've always loved experimenting with my hair ever since I can remember. And today, when fans question me on the street or in their letters, my hair is the single most-often-occurring beauty topic.

As a very little girl, I wore my hair long, about shoulder length, and it was quite curly from the start. I would wear it parted at the side, secured with a barrette, or parted at the center, set and combed into a little pageboy or flip. Sometimes I went to the beauty parlor with my mother, and I even have a vague recollection of her giving me an at-home permanent. I think every mother did that in the "Which twin has the Toni?" era.

By the time I was in grade school, I'd become quite knowledgeable and skilled in dealing with my own hair. Even my mother agreed that I cut it better than the professionals did, and at age twelve or thirteen, my girlfriends were asking me to cut their hair. I suppose I could have

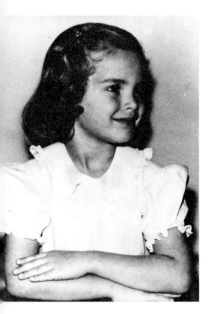

Even when I was a little girl, long, curly hair was one of my favorite looks.

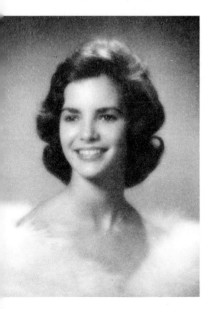

My own variation on the perfect flip, for my high school graduation photo

fallen back on a career in hairdressing if dancing or acting hadn't worked out!

Talk about experimenting! And torture! I went through every phase imaginable—one eye always on the lookout for new hairstyles in fashion and movie magazines.

At one time it was the vogue to set one's hair with socks. You know, the stretchy nylon ones? All my girlfriends and I would turn sections of our hair under, roll them up with the socks and then tie a knot to set the curl. Those rollers were a lot easier to sleep on than the huge brush rollers or soft-drink-can-sized plastic ones I would use to straighten my hair. Not totally in love with my curly hair, I also once tried to chemically straighten it, with less-than-perfect results. I hadn't yet discovered wrapping; nor did I ever hit upon the technique of ironing one's hair on an ironing board. That had to be tricky!

Although I usually kept my hair long, I would try almost anything, and once I chopped it off into a ducktail. Not flat at the nape of the neck like some, but flirty and fluffy all around. I think it was my mother's all-time favorite hairstyle for me. But I let my hair grow out immediately. It was too much of a shock.

There were so many trends! Remember the whole shirtwaist-dress, circle-pin, Pappagallo-shoe, and bubble-cut syndrome? Well, I did have the bubble cut for a while, but I was never too fond of the shirtwaist. And circle pins? Total boredom. I guess it was the first inkling of my rebellious streak. But I did go through the trauma associated with the search for the perfect flip—lightly teased at the crown—as well as the struggles involved in all those complicated "up" hairdos that were popular then.

Elizabeth Taylor's was a sophisticated look I liked, so I even owned a switch (for those of you under twenty-five, that's a ponytail-like hairpiece) that I hardly needed to fill out my already-thick hair. I brushed my hair back from my face, secured it with a headband and then attached the switch at the base of the real ponytail. I piled the whole thing up in a maze of curls and twists and knots, with the mandatory spit curls or sideburns, too. I'll admit it didn't look all that great on me. But Elizabeth Taylor did it, so I thought, why not? At least my hair was off my face.

Another movie star whose look I loved was Audrey Hepburn, especially in *Funny Face.* But struggle and coax as I might, I just couldn't make my curly bangs replicate hers, straight and wispy, brushed to one side across her forehead.

I had much better luck when it came to copying Sandra Dee's hair in those Gidget movies. That was a look I could really relate to. I mean, all that curly hair, pulled into a long, flowing ponytail, with the little waves around the face!

When I think back to the styles I tried, I'm struck with a major difference in hair today: freedom. In those days, there was always one, prevailing, distinct "in" look. But what looks wonderful on someone else may look terrible on you. Today, we're lucky that we have the leeway to find and wear the style or styles that suit us, and that also require minimum maintenance.

WORKING-GIRL HAIR

By the time I came to New York to study acting and dance and audition for Broadway shows, my hair once more was long and slightly curly. Although my first two commercials had nothing at all to do with hair, it was my television commercial for Breck that really started my career rolling. From that Breck-girl exposure I got my first dramatic television role opposite Dennis Weaver on "McCloud."

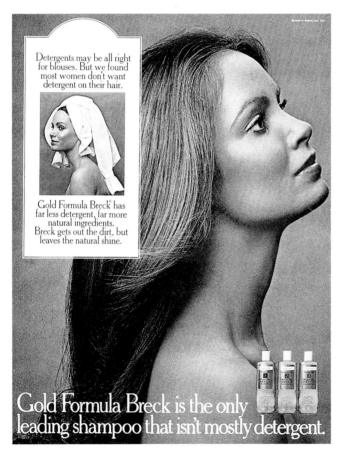

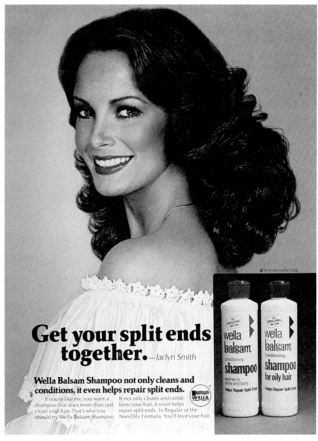

Even as I went into television acting, and eventually to Hollywood, I continued working under contract as a spokeswoman first for Breck, then for the Wella company. For me it wasn't just another acting job. I enjoyed working for companies whose products I really believed in, and actually used.

ANGEL'S HAIR

The hairstyle that Farrah Fawcett wore on "Charlie's Angels" literally created a sensation. But my style attracted a lot of attention, too—so much, in fact, that it became a trap. The producers never wanted to let me change anything about that long, rather perfectly set, curly look because we got so many letters from viewers asking for setting instructions, my haircut tips and all the rest.

In case you've been wondering, here it is. My hair fell well below my shoulders in back, curved to shoulder length in front. The back was left pretty much one length, while the sides were layered all around the face. For the show, I wrapped it to smooth it out; then

As Kelly Garrett in "Charlie's Angels"

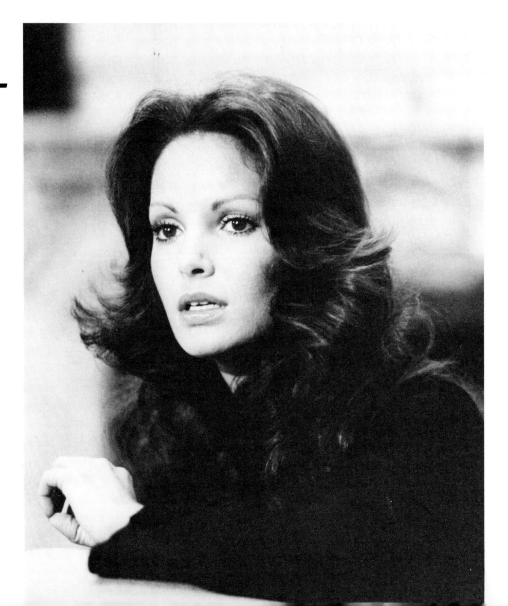

34

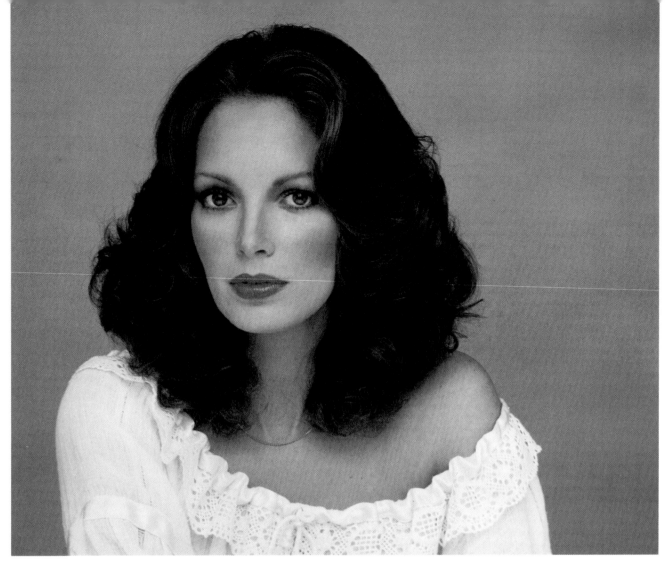

My long, layered Charlie's Angel look

professional hairdressers used electric rollers to set the curl, framing my face, and along the ends. Fortunately, they were adept and became impressively quick at completing this whole process.

For Jaclyn Smith, that hairstyle wasn't very practical. It sometimes fell all over my face while I was writing or eating. But for Kelly Garrett it was perfect, and it looked great on film. It had wonderful body that worked well with all the outdoorsy and windblown activities Kelly was always into.

As much as I liked the way my hair looked on "Charlie's Angels," after five years I began to make subtle changes that were more or less successful. In one episode, I was to have been unwittingly, or at least, unwillingly, drugged with heroin. Since Kelly was supposed to freak out, I decided to show the producers my natural wild, curly/frizzy look. No go. But months later, when we went to Hawaii on location,

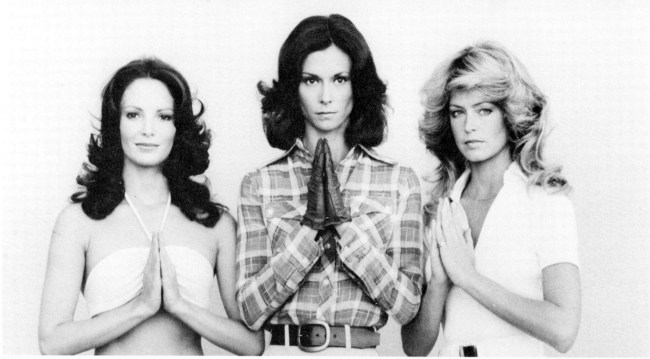

"Charlie's Angels" fans called me "the one with the long brown hair." My first-season partners, Kate Jackson and Farrah Fawcett

The show's success allowed little variation in Kelly's look. My fourth-season "Charlie's Angels" colleagues, Cheryl Ladd and Shelley Hack

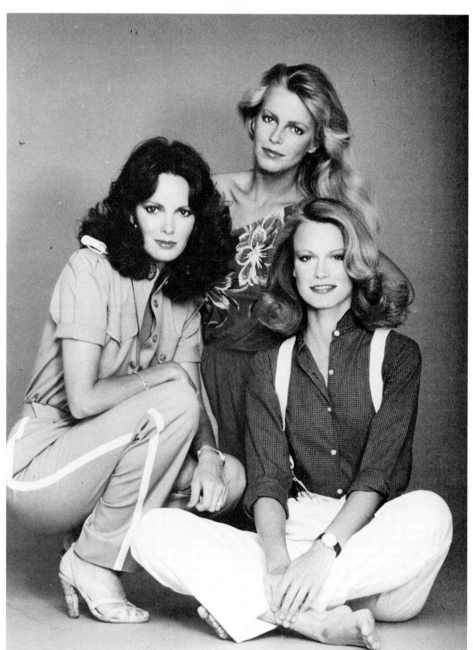

I protested that it was impossible to control my regular style in that kind of humidity. Finally, the powers-that-were accepted a more tamed-down version of my full, curly head.

Toward the end of the final season, my hair was cut slightly shorter and had more allover layers. It was almost the shoulder-length, beveled cut style that I prefer today.

LIFE—AND HAIR—AFTER KELLY GARRETT

With my success pretty well established after "Charlie's Angels," and with an increasing maturity about my looks, I became secure enough to branch out. I was able to avoid becoming a slave to the expected Kelly Garrett look, even knowing how successful it was for me. It was all part of the process we've been talking about: the idea of getting to know and like you as *yourself*—purifying and crystallizing your thoughts about how you look, and how those looks express your true personality. Hair is, of course, only a part of your overall appearance, but I think a woman's hair is highly symbolic of her inner identity. I felt a palpable sense of freedom as I moved on from that Charlie's Angel image. And Lord knows, in a very practical sense, I was happy not to have to re-create that one set look every morning!

As I've noted, my hair is now cut in what is called a beveled cut, a subtle, quarter-inch-at-a-time layering that gives it lots of body and swing. It's essentially normal, thick and curly. But it has straightened considerably since my son was born, which makes it easier to alternate between the frizzy and smooth looks I like.

Care

I usually wash my hair in the shower every morning, with a nondetergent shampoo, in the soft water I insist upon. (We have a water-softening system for the whole house.) Each time I also put on one of several instant conditioners: a liquid protein or one of the several cream conditioners I like. Sometimes I use a cream rinse instead of a conditioner. I switch around like this because I think hair can become immune to a conditioner's benefits if used day after day.

About once a month, I also use a deep-conditioning treatment for hair, using anything from a commercially available protein pack or aloe vera–based product to a do-it-yourselfer like mayonnaise. I'm serious! If there's nothing better on hand, you can just take mayonnaise from the jar, work it into already-wet hair, leave it on for about thirty minutes (standard time for deep-conditioning treatments), then shampoo and rinse well.

With all the nourishing care my hair gets, I do feel the need every once in a while, say, once every two months at least, to get it really squeaky clean and to strip it of any treatment-overload buildup. For that I use a vinegar rinse (see page 44).

You may also want to try a tried-and-true favorite of mine: Nexus Aloe/Rid Clarifier by Jheri Redding.

Styling

Each time I emerge from the shower I have several distinct options before me. I think longer hair, in and of itself, offers versatility, and now, with my noticeably less curly hair, I can choose from a gamut of contemporary styles.

Suppose I want my hair free and curly-to-frizzy, either because my husband always prefers it that way, or because the clothes I'm going to be wearing call for a fuller style. Well, that's the easiest thing to do, since I simply let it dry naturally, arranging the hair a bit with my fingers as the heat lamps in my bathroom gently work out the moisture. I often add a roller or two, along the hairline, to smooth out the front. And that's it.

If I want my hair straight, I wrap it damp. First, I put in two or three rollers, rolled away from my face, at the crown. Then I wrap the neatly combed hair around, using my head as one giant roller. I secure the whole thing with a hair net and begin the drying process that takes from forty-five minutes to an hour. Since my sink is also equipped with a hood-and-hose–type dryer (the kind you can walk around with) I do my makeup or write notes while waiting for my hair to dry. It's worth the time, though, because straight hair is *my* favorite look.

I also have a hand-held dryer, which I use to refine a look: to smooth out pieces in the front of my hair, to tame a wave when I'm going for a straighter style, or, with a natural-bristled, round brush, to turn the ends under.

I've devised all sorts of ways to keep my hair out of my face when I'm most active, that is, playing with my son. I often French-braid it into a single braid down my back. Other times, I just pull it back into a ponytail and secure it with a coated elastic. I have loads of pretty combs and barrettes I use to pull the front and side layers away from my face, allowing the rest to fall free. Pretty ribbons are always appealing, so I often use one to tie a big, romantic, off-center bow—

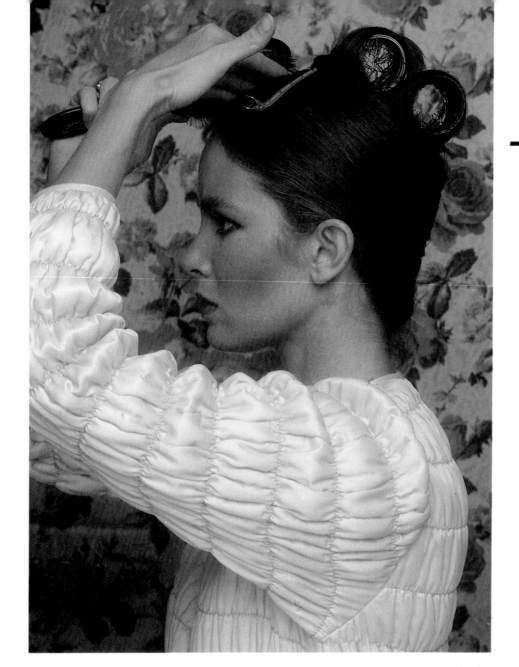

For a smooth style, I wrap and roll my hair damp.

Alice in Wonderland style—that also serves to keep my hair back. One of my favorite "functional" looks is to create that single braid *and* tie a ribbon, or a piece of lace, around my head as a headband.

I sometimes wear my hair up in the evening. And I do like myself with what I consider a Parisian-mannequinesque, slicked-back chignoned look. But my bangs are too short right now to get everything that smooth unless I use a gomina product (hair grease) after straightening it. That's exactly the kind of fussing I don't want to bother with on my own time.

The key, of course, is to take into consideration the kind of clothes

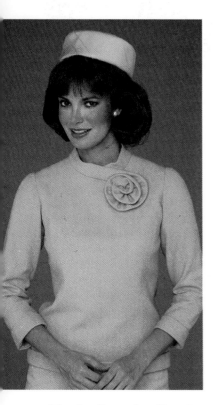

To play Jacqueline Bouvier Kennedy, a three-quarter wig helped achieve a perfect-match hairstyle.

Pinned-on rolls and curls turned me into George Washington's friend Sally Fairfax for TV.

you'll be wearing when you decide on a hairstyle for any given day or evening. Checking out the neckline is not enough. In general, with evening clothes that are a bit bare, I like my hair full and curly. With sweaters and informal daytime clothes, I like it straight.

Behind the Scenes

For films, I study and think through the period my character lives in, as well as consider her age, before selecting the appropriate hairstyle. For instance, on me, straight hair is one way to achieve a very young look.

When I played Jacqueline Bouvier Kennedy, I wore a three-quarter wig, that is, one that starts at the crown. I like to have my own hair exposed around my face and then blended into the wig for a more believable appearance. I don't care what anybody says. *I* can always tell when an actress is wearing a full wig! To get that, or any wig, on

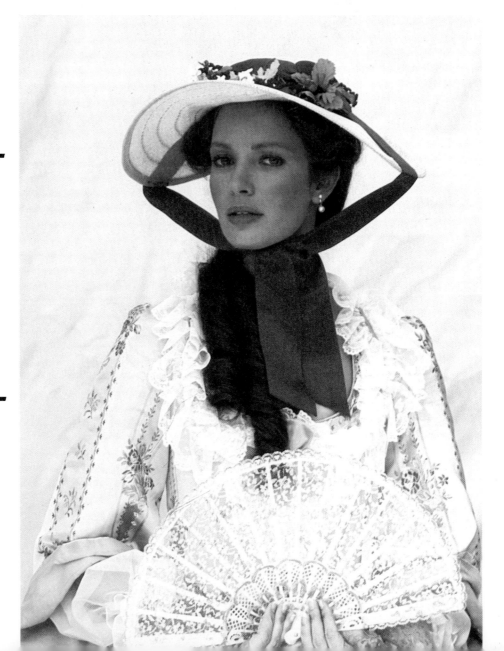

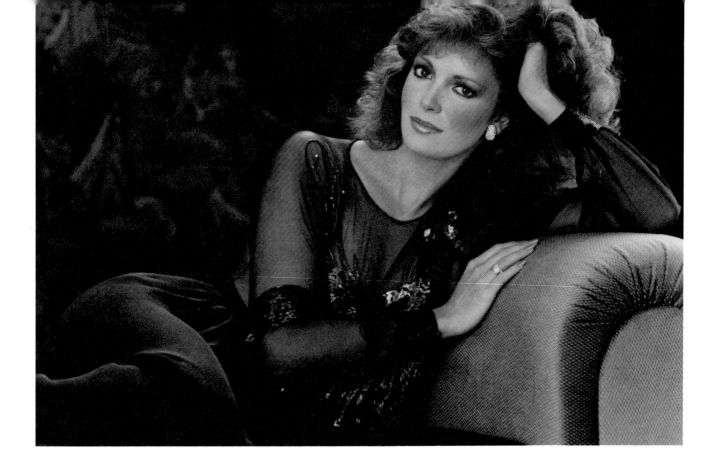

Back to cascading curls for a series of commercials for Max Factor's Epris fragrance

is a bit of a chore. My hair has to be ever-so-neatly pin curled and secured with special flat clips. When the wig first goes on, I think I'm going to have a headache all day. But then I get used to it.

I waste no envy on women of the eighteenth century, if what our research revealed about their hairdos—done for the George Washington film in which I played his first love, Sally Fairfax—is true. Women of that period had seriously "dressed" hair, all piled up into complicated chignons with rolls and curls all over. Apparently they didn't wash those hairstyles for months! And all the powder they put on their hair!

The women and the men of that period also wore wigs. But it was my own hair you saw on Sally, although it did have a rather interesting system of sausagelike rolls and spit curls and little packages of curls attached. The resulting look was quite beautiful, but it ruled out my habitual midday catnap at the studio. I couldn't put my head down to rest without the risk of having to reconstruct this coiffure before afternoon shooting began.

Even though I haven't played her for years, I wore a variation of the Kelly Garrett look for a recent series of Epris perfume commercials for Max Factor. My hair was first set with those old-fashioned sponge rollers when it was still damp from washing or lightly spritzed with water. When it dried, the stylist used a special crimping iron that made sort of zigzag dents in my hair for a very modern look. The finished result was full hair with lots of interesting texture, but still under control.

Color

Along with the rest of the female population of America, I've been known to take advantage of a sunny day and squeeze a bit of fresh lemon juice on my hair before going outdoors to encourage my naturally blond highlights. Having been rather pleased with my chestnut brown hair all my life (no, I wasn't one of those teenagers who experimented with peroxide), I've never been tempted to drastically alter its color. However, for my work in front of the camera, I do need to highlight it a bit because even my medium-brown shade registers as black on film.

Since spending time in a hair salon is about the last thing I want to do on a fifteen-to-eighteen-hour shooting day, I have my one-process highlighting done on the set or at home. (In two-process color, the hair is first bleached of its natural pigment, then tinted.) I get most of my haircuts on the set or at home, too. In any case, I think my highlights look natural because they're actually done in several golden shades, subtly woven into my own hair, just in front, where the sun would lighten it anyway.

My first gray hair didn't alarm me as much as you might think, because it showed up under unusual circumstances. Years ago, I was hit in the head with a rock—a long and boring story—and then was reinjured in the same spot, shooting an especially action-packed scene for "Charlie's Angels." The hair that regrew in that area was sparser than the rest, and suddenly began to sprout the odd gray hair.

When I started to see the more predictable grays at the temple—and this isn't a big problem for me, yet!—I just thought, Hey, these look like highlights. I like them.

Don't get me wrong. I don't fancy myself with steely gray hair. At the very least, it might limit my range of acting roles. But for the time being, I can simply camouflage any that turn up with the blond highlights.

I'm not so concerned about the future, either. There are so many good hair-coloring products available now for both at-home and salon application. Hair coloring doesn't carry the damage potential it used to. In fact, many current products and processes can actually improve the condition of your hair.

• Many people have asked me about how to find hair-color and styling pros they can deal with and, most important of all, whose work they can trust. I don't think that's an easy task for any woman, and for me, it's critical. In my business, these experts have to do work you admire, and you have to really get along well. On a picture, you're going to be together for up to eighteen hours a day. You're practically living together; the trusted pros become your friends.

But finding and working with someone new is always tricky. I don't want to smother all of the stylist's creative impulses, but on the other hand, I can't let a hairdresser go wild. It's still *my* hair, *my* fashion shoot or ad. And believe me, I do know my hair better than anyone else.

• It's just as important for each of you to discover a professional hair stylist with whom you can "live," even if you're only going to visit the salon once every two months or so. When you're contemplating

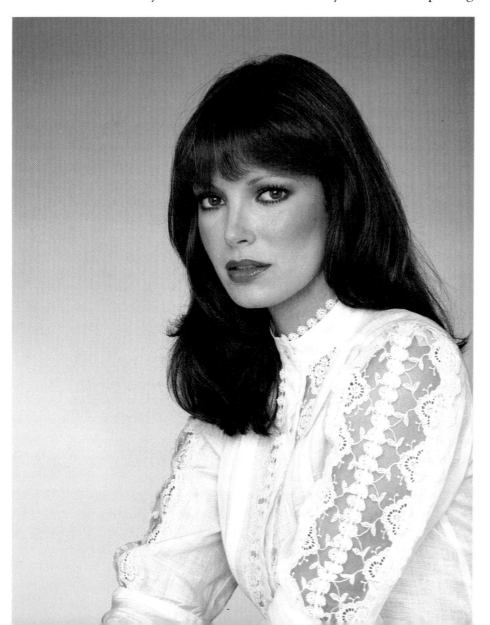

JACLYN SMITH'S HAIR-CARE GUIDE

The Basics

- Daily washing with a nondetergent shampoo.

- Next, an instant conditioner formulated for your hair type and its current "status."

- Long hair needs a quick cream rinse for detangling.

- Comb—don't brush—wet hair. Style.

The Extras

- Once-a-month deep conditioning with a commercial, leave-in product, or simply, mayonnaise from the jar.

- Once every two months, a thorough cleansing to remove all treatment buildup. My recipe:
  ½ cup white vinegar
  added to
  1 quart boiling water.
  Let solution cool.
  Apply to just-washed hair.
  Finish with a cool to ice-cold rinse.

- A little lemon juice, when in the sun, for natural highlights.

---

a cut, that essential element in overall hair appearance, ask for a consultation before you commit to an expensive appointment.

In talking just for a few minutes with a hair expert, you can sense whether he or she is someone who understands, and will heed, your wishes. Feel free to look elsewhere if the vibes just aren't right.

- If you like what the pro is suggesting, in terms of the cut or even coloring, give him or her a chance. Depending on the current condition and length of your hair, it may take several visits, and therefore, several months, to achieve the agreed-upon color or cut.

Also, don't expect any cut to hold forever. The shorter your hair, the more often you will have to go back to refresh its line. If you wait too long, your hair will sort of "forget" and get raggedy and shapeless, even if the original cut was superb.

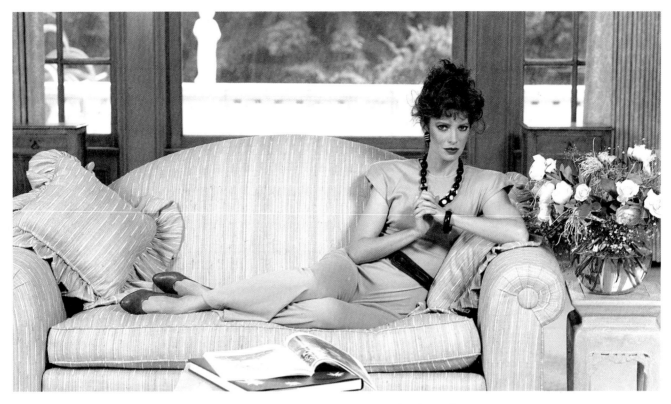

- Remember to take into consideration your head-to-toe look, when you and the stylist discuss your cut. The wrapper-shrouded shoulders and attached head reflected in the salon mirror just won't do. Stand up so that the stylist can assess the overall effect. You suggest it, if he or she doesn't.

- Many women make the mistake of fighting their hair's natural tendencies. Yes, I myself will spend up to an hour straightening my hair. But I've also learned to have it cut and styled according to its true texture.

- Do ask the professional stylist to show you how to deal with your hair at home. There's nothing worse than feeling alone, helpless and inept, facing freshly washed, just-cut hair.

    When I travel on the job, I'm usually lucky enough to have a good hairstylist around. But it's comforting to know I can handle my hair (quite well, thank you) myself.

- There's no one hairstyle that's going to suit you for a lifetime. Your face, your taste in clothes, your life-style—everything—changes.

So should your hair. Some women who are old enough to know better seem to stick with a look that's old-fashioned or patently too young for them. I often think it has to do with trying to hold on to an earlier, happier time. But you can't take your college-yearbook picture with you through life; you must allow your self-image to grow with you.

• As for hair color, I think shading hair a little lighter is usually more natural than making it darker, and more flattering as we age. Whether yours is one- or two-process color, never allow your hair to become all one color, one solid shade. There's nothing more unnatural than one-tone black or blond hair.

• I'm not a ravenous consumer of hair spray, but I do like to have it around, especially for those nights I decide to wear my hair up. Just a smidgen, sprayed onto a cotton ball and then dabbed on the hair, works wonders in taming and "gluing up" those straggling wisps. Plus, you have pinpoint control this way.

• Sometimes I add heat to my deep-conditioning routine by—are you ready for this?—going outside into the sunshine. My hair just looks like an intended wet-look hairdo, and the sun seems to help the conditioner penetrate more deeply and fully. Meanwhile, I can work in the garden or play with my son.

• I can't stand it when my hair doesn't shine. So, when my hair has been overworked or made dull by the water in a foreign country, I sometimes rub a little hairdressing between my palms and work it lightly through my hair. You know that old saying, "A little dab'll do ya." Well, that's the idea, unless, of course, you're going for a wet-look style, which can be quite attractive.

• If I only get one message across here, it's that we're so lucky to be women in *this* era. To be considered "with it" today, you don't need to wear layered false eyelashes, drawn-on eyeliner, or teased-up hair. *Natural* is the beauty attitude today, which means you can wear your hair any way that's flattering to you—permed, straight, curly, short, long, layered, or blunt-cut. *Any* way! It's all *in*. Given all this freedom and versatility, isn't it foolish to waste a lot of time fussing with your hair? Just think of all the other wonderful ways you can spend that time!

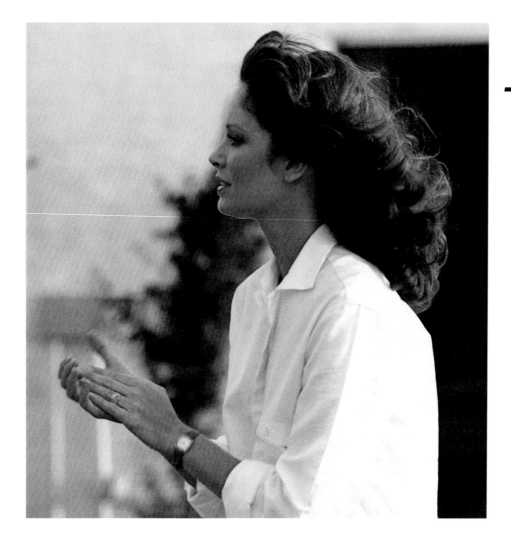

Calling the dogs for a run after a day on the set of **Night Kill** *(1980). My "naturally" glossy head of hair actually takes a lot of work.*

CONVERSATION WITH AN EXPERT: EMMA DI VITTORIO ON HAIR CONDITION AND COLOR

Emma Di Vittorio began her career as a professional in hair care and styling with the famous House of Westmore, beauty salon to the stars during Hollywood's studio-system heyday. For the last two decades, she has worked free-lance in movies and television. I met Emma about seven years ago on "Charlie's Angels," and we've since become devoted co-workers as well as friends. Here, Emma and I talk about tried-and-true methods for keeping hair in great condition and choosing its most flattering color.

JS: Emma, what's your basic recipe for good, consistent hair care?

EDV: Well, I believe in washing the hair as often as possible—not to mention as often as needed—to keep it very clean and glossy. That can mean every day, even with naturally dry hair, if it's conditioned properly each time.

JS: How does a woman know what shampoo and what sort of conditioner is right for her?

EDV: There's always the trial-and-error approach to arriving at the products that work for you, that give the results you're looking for. Or, for a shortcut, you could visit a professional hairdresser and get guidance as to the types of products to look for.

One thing I've noticed is that the best day-after-day, year-after-year results seem to be achieved when your hair-care products are alternated or rotated. I can't say why this is so; it's just been my experience.

Also, it's important to remember that your hair, which I call a barometer of what's going on in the body, changes with certain other influences. So if you go on a drastic diet, change climates or begin taking significant medication, you may well have to adjust your hair-care regime accordingly. Again, I think a pro could save you a lot of time in making the proper adjustments.

JS: I know you particularly like natural products or those with natural ingredients. Why?

EDV: I just think that among the best shampoos and conditioners I've worked with, those with wheat germ oil, aloe vera, or uncolored henna are truly excellent. After all, these are ingredients that have been proved—for centuries!

As we both learned, working on the "George Washington" miniseries, in Revolutionary times they even used bear grease to condition their hair. And I'm intrigued with the new products containing jojoba oil. I also wonder if, someday, the super proteins of tofu might not make for good hair treatments.

JS: You recommend washing hair often and using an instant conditioner each time. What about deep conditioners, the kind you leave on, sometimes with a heat cap?

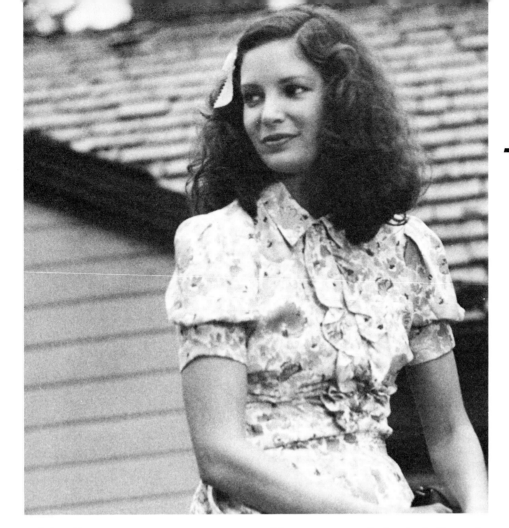

My hair's natural waves came in handy when I played the young Jacqueline Bouvier.

EDV: I'm not a great supporter of heat caps and don't believe in leaving anything on the hair for more than about fifteen or twenty minutes. By that time, whatever conditioning benefits there are have been achieved. And besides, I'm wary of allowing hair to stay wet for too long. I learned in motion-picture work in which scenes with wet hair had to be repeated again and again, for days, that the actress's hair really seemed weakened from the experience.

JS: What about injecting a cream rinse into your regular clean-and-care regimen?

EDV: Cream rinse is fine for hair that tangles easily and for people with very sensitive scalps, especially little girls with long, fine hair. But since these rinses are based largely on wax, they do sometimes have a buildup effect. On the other hand, there's certainly nothing harmful in them. It's just that they should never be confused with, and substituted for, a conditioner.

JS: What are the right hair tools for gentle care?

EDV: Combing gently, working from the ends upward, is absolutely the way to deal with wet hair. And I'm talking about a relatively wide-toothed, nonmetallic comb. The only exception I can think of is Mason Pearson's detangling brush with widely spaced bristles that act like three or four combs going at once.

For styling and arranging dry hair, I recommend rubber- or plastic-bristled brushes. To finish, to polish the hair, you might want to work with a natural-bristled brush for just a minute or two, because they tend to smooth the hair cuticles and make it shine.

JS: Does summer or vacation-time exposure to sun, and swimming, have any negative effects on hair's condition?

EDV: My many years of living and working in California have proved it does. Hair ought to be protected from the sun just the way your skin is. For instance, even uncolored hair can get brassy or fade from constant exposure to bright sunlight. Wearing a hat and/or wearing a conditioning gel in the hair—you know, for a sort of wet look—are really important if you're going to be sitting on a beach. And I always recommend that a woman wash her hair—wash, not just rinse—every time she comes out of a chlorinated pool or the ocean.

JS: How do you feel about the use of hair spray?

EDV: Sometimes it's the only thing that'll keep hair in place, the way you want it. But there are other options, like the newer styling gels, that are less harsh on the hair.

JS: What should come first, a new haircut or hair coloring?

EDV: I think cut, because that's the foundation for everything about the finished look.

JS: Is there anyone who should never consider hair coloring?

EDV: Well, in film and TV work, I've seen every type of hair colored. It's such an individual thing. Of course, if you have fine, thin hair and put on a thirty-volume peroxide with a booster and leave it on for two hours, you're going to wreck your hair.

On the other hand, color processes have been made so much gentler that old taboos like never coloring permed hair are no longer valid.

JS: What's the safest hair-coloring process?

EDV: In the hands of an experienced professional, anything is "safe." But using hennas is undeniably least harmful to the hair itself. And with colored hennas, you can get marvelous shades of bronze, golden blond and mahogany for red hair. I'm quite a fan of henna for coloring.

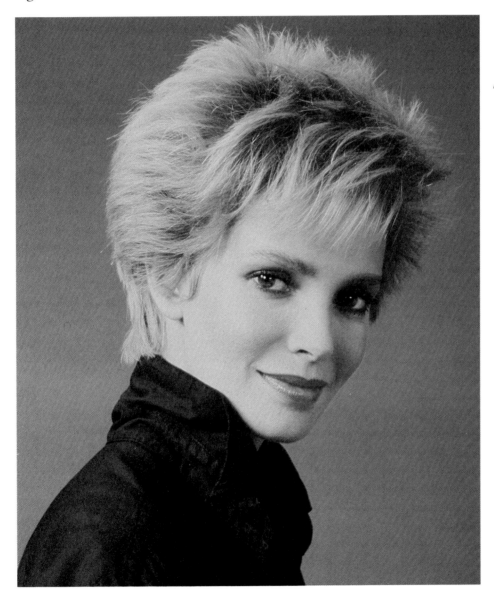

I got the chance to become a cropped blonde for **Always.**

Otherwise, except if you're going for a dramatic change, especially going lighter, you would want to use a one-process color, where the tint is simply deposited in the hair. For those more dramatic changes, you have to have a two-process color—that is when the hair is first stripped of its natural color, then the desired shade is put on.

JS: How can a woman test a contemplated hair color without committing herself to it?

EDV: There do exist overnight, wash-out colorings and spray-in products that we use a lot on the set, to match a double's hair to the star's. But they don't yield particularly natural-looking results. I honestly think the best way to "try on" a new hair color is to check yourself out in a wig of the proposed shade.

JS: Should a woman who's never colored her hair do it at the first signs of gray hair?

EDV: Obviously that's a matter of individual choice. There's no need to be afraid of damage from hair color as there used to be in the past. In my opinion, even just a few gray hairs in otherwise dark hair often make too dramatic a contrast; the gray calls too much attention to itself. And it is usually easily covered with one-process coloring.

But on fairer, golden blond or lightest brown hair, sometimes the gray can look like white-blond streaks and can be quite pretty.

JS: Should eyebrows be dyed to match a new hair color?

EDV: I wouldn't say so. My theory is not to mess with them, unless they're very dark and the hair's very blond. But in general, hair color and brow color don't have to match perfectly.

JS: What should a woman do if she's unhappy with the results of a professional-salon coloring job?

EDV: I'd say, in the situation you propose, that the woman should return to the same colorist. I'll tell you why. If indeed the pro has made a mistake, he or she has still learned a lot about your hair and how it reacts. I'd give the original colorist a second chance.

I should add, though, that it isn't fair to make your final judgment about new hair coloring for at least twenty-four hours, including at least one shampoo. The color continues to oxidize a bit, even after you've left the salon, and needs time to settle. With really drastic changes in color, I'd say wait a week before deciding you don't like it, or contemplating any alteration in the color.

JS: You're obviously biased in favor of professional hair coloring. Do you truly believe women can't color their own hair successfully at home?

EDV: I don't believe most of them have the experience to do as good a job as a salon colorist. I mean, a pro can tell when he or she is mixing up a batch of a specific coloring product if this batch is slightly different, and make the adjustments necessary. Trained hair colorists know about how coloring done in an air-conditioned salon, or in an overheated room, can affect the process. It's a sensitivity that can only be gained with years of experience.

Hair coloring is a delicate and complex process. And as I say, you only have one head of hair. You can't put it in the closet and pull out another one!

JS: What is the biggest problem you see with women who have their hair colored?

EDV: I think it's a problem of attitude. Many women who have had their hair colored seem to think, Well, it's done. My hair's perfect now. I don't have to touch it. They forget that hair care is more important than ever—to keep it looking as good as it did the moment they came out of the salon. Some women give up responsibility for their hair's condition. But the hairdresser can't follow you home, except in the movies. Remember *Shampoo!*

CONVERSATION WITH AN EXPERT: STEPHEN KNOLL ON HAIRCUT AND STYLING

Stephen Knoll is a free-lance hair stylist who left the Midwest eleven years ago to land his first job at the famed Manhattan hair salon Kenneth's. He added to his top-flight experience with stints at Saks Fifth Avenue's salon and the Pierre Michel salon, before work with a fashion photographer established him as one of the most sought-after hairdressers for print ad, fashion layout and commercial work. I first met Stephen when we did a TV Guide *cover shoot*

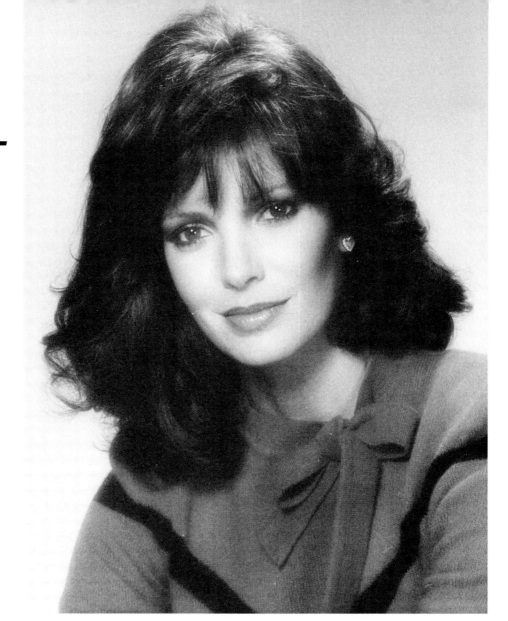

together about two years ago, and we have often worked together on commercials and fashion layouts. Stephen and I talk about the ways to a good cut and personal styling in the '80s.

JS: It seems to me that we've moved away from the supremacy of the finished style, putting more emphasis today on haircut and condition. Do you agree?

SK: Absolutely. The condition of the hair is critical, because, like a painter, you have to have a good canvas to start with. But I'd say that today, the cut is *as* important as the hair's condition. You can't just have a good cut and dried-out hair. Nor can you have luxurious, wonderfully conditioned hair with a horrible cut. Both are disasters.

But the big change is the fact that stylists, and women themselves, aren't relying on just the final styling to make everything look wonderful. They know how crucial cut and condition are.

JS: Can you categorize the kinds of cuts that work best for specific hair types? What approach makes sense for straight, fine hair, for instance?

SR: Taking into account the vast differences in individuals, I still think you can say that fine, straight hair is best with a blunt cut. If the hair is straight, but heavier, you can vary the approach more. You could layer the front a bit, have blunt-cut bangs or layer the entire head.

JS: What about fine or thin hair that has some wave?

SK: In that case, I definitely wouldn't recommend allover layers, but more of a tapered cut to reduce the weight of the hanging hair and encourage volume and the natural wave pattern.

JS: How about thick, wavy hair?

SK: Basically, I think layering here is the best way to use the hair's fullness and to give the woman an easy-to-care-for look.

JS: Can hair that's very curly—even frizzy—still be fine?

SK: Sure. The texture of the hair has nothing to do with its volume, or the amount you have on your head. You can have fine, curly hair or coarse, curly hair.

JS: Okay then, what cutting technique would you use on fine, curly hair?

SK: Generally speaking, it's got to be a good all-around cut, cut where the hair is about the same length from the scalp all over. But that's not to say it will necessarily fall all to one length.

JS: Thick, curly hair?

SK: I'd go to one extreme or the other with this type of hair. Either it should be long and full, or definitely short. In-between lengths tend to make for a round-headed, bushy look that's really no look at all.

JS: You mentioned a painter's canvas earlier. What about tools?

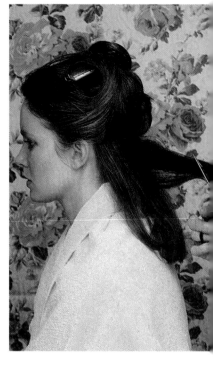

Getting a beveled cut—a series of quarter-inch layers—perfect for thick, wavy hair

SK: I always use professional haircutting scissors, never a razor. A razor slices the hair at an angle, leaving it much more susceptible to splitting and breaking off. I'm not convinced that any woman can be great at cutting her own hair, but if she does, she must use haircutting scissors. I've found women who use their nail scissors to trim their bangs!

JS: What considerations go into choosing the right cut?

SK: Everything from allover body size to hair type. A woman five feet ten inches who's not thin might still have very refined facial features that tempt her to try a very short hair cut. But her overall size dictates more hair, so she doesn't end up looking like a pinhead. The stylist has to look at the whole individual as a three-dimensional being. A cut that's great from the front might not flatter the profile at all. It's got to be a complete picture.

JS: A lot of women wonder if there's an age limit for having long hair.

SK: I've never believed in limitations imposed because of age. A woman could look her best in shoulder-length hair at fifty, if the hair's color, cut and her own face and figure were in harmony.

JS: Does hair grow more or faster if it's cut often? Or is that a myth?

SK: It just seems that way. Women who have hair coloring can tell you that your hair grows about the same amount every month, barring a big change in hormones, or medications, or some other factors. They can tell by how regularly their roots have to be retouched.

The advantage of regular haircuts, or trims, is that they keep the ends neat, discouraging splitting and breakage. I think that even if a woman is trying to let her hair grow out, she should have her hair cut about every five or six weeks.

JS: Can a certain haircut serve to hide or distract from a less attractive area of the face, or from a less-than-perfect feature?

SK: Hair can play a big role in detracting from faults. For instance, for a thick neck or double chin, you'd want the hair much fuller on top of the head and around the eyes, or quite long. You wouldn't want the hair cropped at the jawline. Obviously, for an elegant, thin

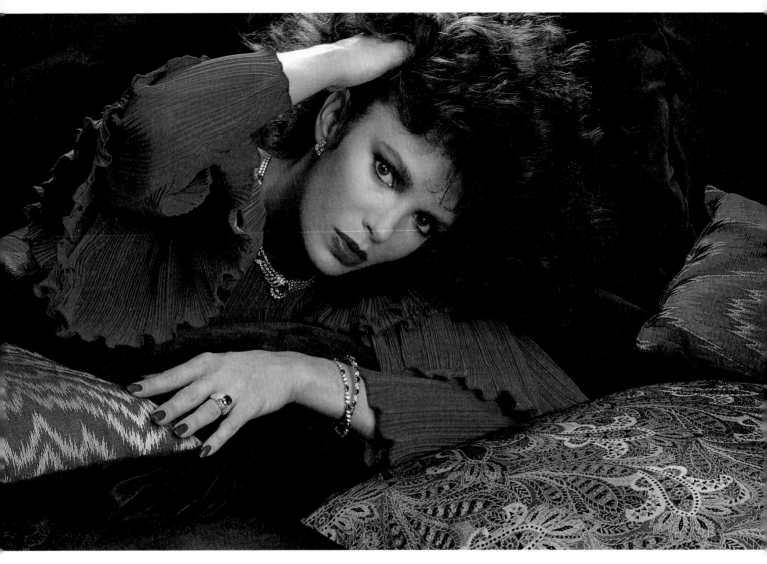

neck, hair cut just to the jawline is great. And as an aside, I'd note the importance of an attractive hairline if you're contemplating one of the currently fashionable short cuts that reveal the nape of the neck.

It's interesting that for a narrow or broad forehead, the haircutting solution is the same: bangs or fringe. It's just that for a very narrow forehead, you'd start the bangs further back in the hair, to give the illusion of length and balance.

JS: What if a woman has a large nose she'd like to de-emphasize?

SK: Well, I happen to like large, strong noses. But if you want to distract from one, you'd usually opt for a style with plenty of volume. Not a severe, geometric cut.

JS: What do you think is the biggest mistake women make in selecting a haircut or style?

SK: I think many women are resistant to change. They don't realize that with the passage of time, after a diet or a weight gain, or just if they've had the same exact look for three years, it's time to move on.

JS: But how do you find the right hairdresser for that change? Should you look for someone new, even if you're happy with the stylist you've been going to for years?

SK: In most cases, women find a good stylist by word-of-mouth, from talking with their women friends. If you're contemplating a pretty drastic change, I'd ask for a consultation before the big cut, so that you and the hairdresser can see if you understand each other and agree on what would be best.

And yes, even though you're happy with your stylist, it may be that he or she knows you *too* well. Perhaps he or she can no longer look at you with a fresh eye or see you in a new and different light. So I do believe in going to a new person and trying out a new approach to your appearance, even if your best-ever look is left behind. Change for change's sake is liberating. Plus, you can always go back to your all-time-favorite look later on.

JS: How do you respond to a woman who brings you a picture from a fashion or a beauty magazine to show the cut she wants?

SK: In principle, it's not a bad idea. But in my experience, a woman usually brings a photo of a girl twenty to thirty years younger than she, with wavy, thick hair, when she herself has bone-straight hair. But at least it gives the stylist a starting point, a notion of what the woman expects. Though the stylist may have to gently dissuade or ultimately disappoint the client, they have a point of discussion anyway.

One thing to keep in mind, too, is that—as you well know—for fashion and advertising photos we often do things with the hair in the studio that aren't replicable for real-life, on-the-street wear. For a professional shoot, I often have to do something dramatic, with clips or props or whatever, to make the hair look right at that moment.

And many times, the hair I'm working with isn't really capable of achieving the required style without these extras.

JS: In general, what are the trends in hairstyles today?

SK: Well, the great leap forward over the last ten years or so is that women don't want to fight their hair's natural tendencies so much. They realize that working well with what's there, that is, working through cut and conditioning, can give them a flattering, modern, easy-to-care-for style that makes sense. Especially now that women are so active, in business, sports, everything!

In a more specific sense, anything that is too set-looking, too precise and structured is passé, I think. To me, that hair have shine and movement is everything. That's why I'm not so crazy about hair ornaments and combs and things.

JS: You mean you're against anything in the hair?

SK: Well, sometimes a soft ribbon or bow, or tying it up with a scarf. But I love the fluidity of well-cared-for hair and don't think you should constrict that with anything stiff like combs and barrettes. Then the hair can't move in one continuous shape, the way it will with a good cut.

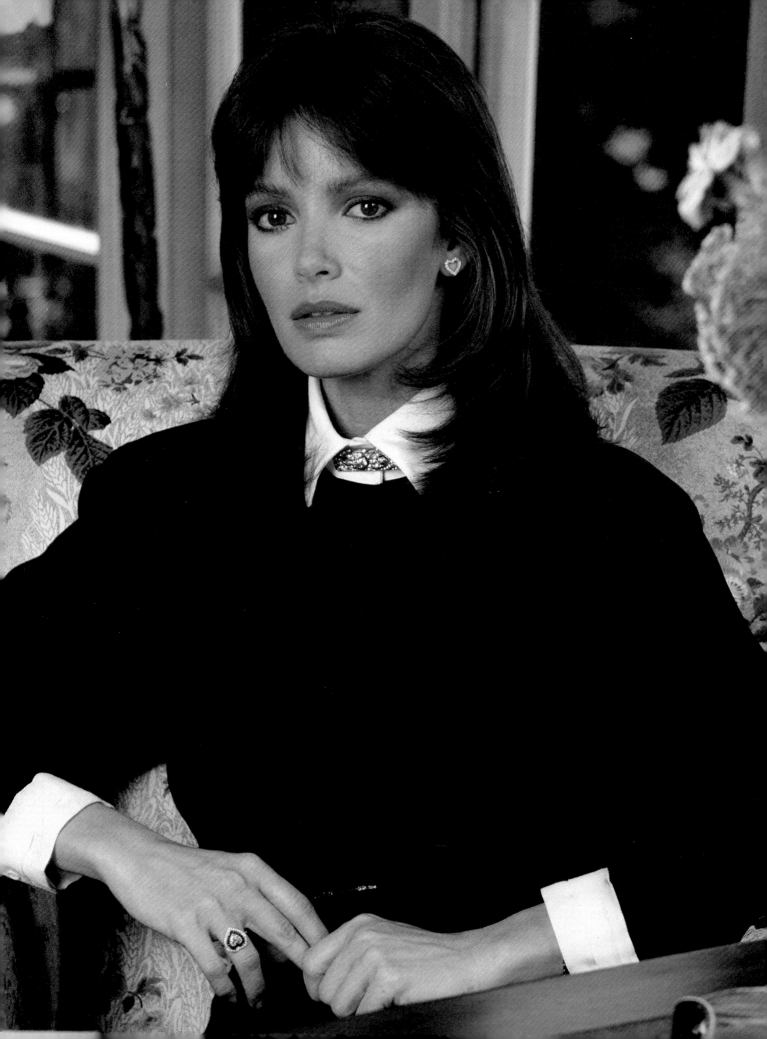

CHAPTER 4

You've Only Got One Skin: Make It Beautiful

Of course there are many women, even famous actresses, successful performers *and* models, who don't have perfect skin. But no matter what sort of skin you've been born with—heredity has so much to do with it, I think—there's really no excuse for abusing it or allowing it to be less an asset than it can be. Think of it this way. It's your body's largest and most visible organ; it's your wrapping, your protection. It really deserves your attention, don't you agree?

I'm certainly not the first person you've heard *this* from: good skin care has to be a routine part of your beauty life, as automatic as brushing your teeth.

I wasn't much interested in a complex skin-care ritual when I was a teenager. (I'm still not!) Blessed with untroubled, basically combination skin, I was simply concerned with its being clean. Particularly when I had to wear makeup for stage performances, I couldn't wait to wash it all off when I got home. Thoroughly cleaning my face before bed was an addiction; I just liked my face to look and feel clean.

I didn't use moisturizer then, and, I hate to admit, I never thought about a sunscreen either. Luckily I've never been one of those people who can bear lying out in the sun, baking, for very long. I wasn't aware of protecting my skin, and I surely liked being tan. But most sun exposure then, as now, took place while I was doing something else: swimming, running, walking, whatever. I think I inadvertently avoided a lot of possible damage simply because I got too bored just sunbathing.

SKIN CARE: A.M. AND P.M.

Not surprisingly, through my years of commercials, stage and film work, I've developed quite a routine, that automatic-pilot approach to taking care of my skin.

I wake up with basically clean skin, so in my shower, I merely steam my face and rinse with hot, then cold water. I don't feel the need for soap at this point.

Next, I smooth on a little mild astringent lotion or a skin freshener with a piece of cotton. Then moisturizer. I have favorite moisturizers of differing weights that I alternate among, depending on how my skin looks and feels, the time of year and the weather. Adjustments have to be made for, say, the humidity of Houston, when I go home for a visit.

At night before bed, I first remove any makeup thoroughly with Albolene cream. However, I also use liquid eye-makeup remover because the rich cream sometimes leaves a film over my eyes—something I find highly annoying when I get in bed to read or occasionally watch television.

To remove any last traces of makeup and the cream, I follow up with a dry-skin soap and water, first hot and then a cool splash. Afterward, a mild astringent and then a moisturizer. If I have any blemishes—yes, movie stars do get an occasional pimple, too—I apply a drying lotion or other topical medicine prescribed by my dermatologist.

As you can see, it's all really quite simple and not overly time-consuming. I happen to pick and choose among products I've used for years, mixed in with the newer ones I've discovered. I suppose the whole idea of a day-in, day-out skin regimen would be even easier if you choose a one-brand system that's all spelled out for you, step-by-step. The real key is to do it—every morning and every night.

JACLYN SMITH'S ALL-STAR SKIN-CARE REGIMEN

To me, the critical time for your skin is before bed. Here is my step-by-step approach to keeping it superclean and healthy.

P.M. Regimen

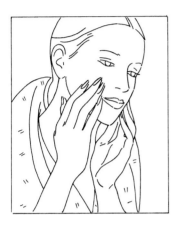

1. Remove *all* of the day's makeup with a gentle cream; use a nongreasy liquid remover for getting off every last trace of eye makeup.

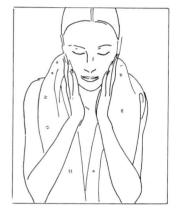

2. Wash with a soap formulated for your skin type; rinse first with hot, then cool water.

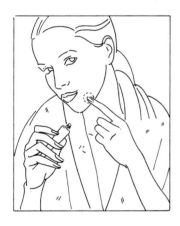

3. Apply a drying lotion to any apparent blemish or pimple.

4. Get plenty of sleep!

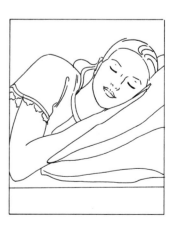

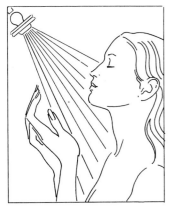

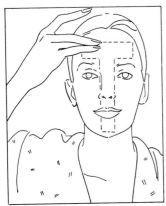

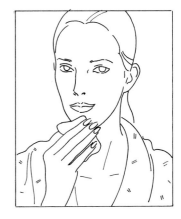

1. Since you awaken with essentially clean skin, your morning, premakeup work is minimal. Start by steaming your face in your morning shower or bath. Rinse, again with hot water followed by cold.

2. Using a cotton ball, go over your face with an astringent, for oily skins, or a light tonic or freshener.

3. Apply a moisturizer formulated for your skin type. You might need two: a rich one for dry areas; a particularly light one for the T-zone, oily sections. But all of your face needs some rehydrating.

TREATS AND TREATMENTS

Aside from the daily habit of good skin care, there are, of course, every-once-in-a-while things you can, and should, do to keep your face looking its best: *before* the makeup goes on.

- For instance, I often lubricate my eyelashes before I go to sleep. I know it sounds funny, but your lashes can become more lustrous with a little conditioning, just as your hair can. With my fingertips or a cotton swab, I simply smooth on a little castor oil or a product called Talika, a Vaseline-like cream specifically formulated for treating the lashes.

- I try to have a deep-cleansing and moisturizing facial once a month at the very least. But the more hectic my work schedule, the more a professional facial can help; sometimes I treat my face two or three times a month.

Even though I know from experience how much an aesthetician can do to keep my skin glowing, I still think having a facial is a bit of a luxury. I suppose it's because anything so enjoyable, so soothing and relaxing seems almost sinful—like having a whole bowl of caviar to yourself!

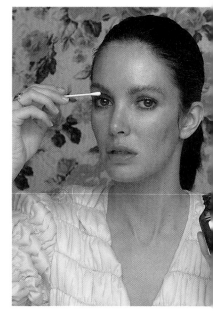

Eyelashes benefit from conditioning just as hair does.

- Serious skin problems should be taken immediately to a dermatologist. I'm not the kind of woman who likes or needs to fill up her day with appointments with this doctor and that specialist. Nonetheless, I have learned the value of establishing a relationship with a qualified dermatologist, if only to check things from time to time.

  Except for one emotionally traumatic period, just after my grandfather died, I've never had to consult a doctor for skin problems. I just visit my dermatologist about once every six to eight months to confirm that I'm maintaining my complexion correctly, and often, to discuss products with him.

- I've added a lip emollient to my regular collection of skin-care products. I use it at night or during the day, whenever I think about it. If I forget, the dry, chapped feeling my lips get will eventually remind me to smooth some on.

- Traveling requires some adjustments, even additions to your regular at-home skin-care regimen. For example, if I'm on location someplace warm and dry, like Arizona, I'll create my own moisturizing facial. I just slather on the Albolene cream, and while I'm in my hot bath, rest for a while with a warm washcloth over my face.

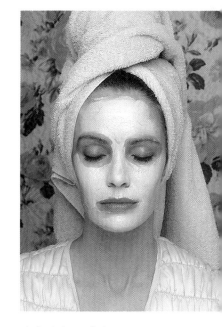

A facial mask is a wonderful once-a-week soother for the skin.

- At home, I take full advantage, at least once a week, of the effective moisturizing masks commercially available as well as the whipped-up versions of my own on occasion. When it's avocado season in California, I love nothing better than a mashed-avocado mask (warmed over the double boiler) during my bath. Talk about getting back to nature!

- I wish I were the sort of person who's organized enough to have all her skin-care preparations neatly poured into plastic travel bottles, but I'm not. I do double up on skin-care-product purchases, however, so that, along with my makeup, I can have a travel kit ready to go at all times, with no annoying disappointments about having forgotten a favorite product.

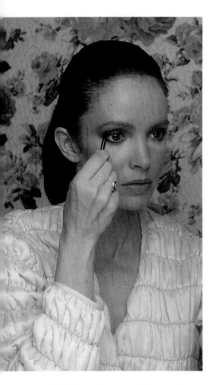

Tidying brows is best done, and least painful, **before** *my morning shower.*

There is also the fact (the rationalization?) that my trips are often long ones—with the weeks of rehearsal, wardrobe and actual shooting that go into a movie. So those cute, small-sized travel containers wouldn't necessarily hold enough cream or lotion to cover me for the entire stay.

- I've discovered that, for some reason, plucking my eyebrows is best done in the morning, before my shower. That way, any puffiness or redness has a chance to subside during the shower itself.

- I also sometimes use those special facial-scrub pads. They work great as exfoliators, removing the top layer of dead skin cells. But you have to be very careful and be sure not to overscrub, which can cause damage or irritation.
  I don't usually include a cream with beauty grains in it in my own regimen, but one can also be used—perhaps more gently than scrub pads, depending on the smoothness of the grains—to achieve exfoliation. You really have to work with either method for a while to determine whether once-a-day or once-a-week use is for you.

- Maybe it's because I don't smoke and only rarely have a glass of wine with dinner, but I'm not often troubled with eye redness. However, when I'm tired, makeup artists have sometimes put drops in my eyes, especially before a still close-up. Many actresses and models use them regularly to put a little extra sparkle in their eyes as well as to combat redness.

- A great summertime refresher for your face as well as your spirits is a trick I learned behind the scenes. After I've been under the brutally hot lights of a film set, the makeup artist will take a refrigerator-chilled mild astringent, like Sea Breeze, and use it to dampen a chamois cloth (that's also been stored in the fridge) to freshen my forehead, neck and wrists. It feels wonderful!

SUN SENSE

Nobody loves sunshine more than I do. But we've all become increasingly aware of its aging effects on skin. As I've told you, I was never much of a dedicated sun worshiper, but I do like to have a little healthy color. And living where I do, I couldn't avoid exposure to the sun if I wanted to. After all, part of the joy of living in California is playing and working outdoors, all year round.

I enjoy having a slight golden tan on my body and legs. But I'm very strict with myself when it comes to sun on my face. I realize that some facial lines and wrinkles are inevitable, but why do anything to *encourage* them?

So these days, after applying moisturizer, which used to be the finale of my skin-care program, I've added an important step: sunscreen. I use it every day, even if I'm only planning to be in the yard with Gaston and then do a few errands.

In truth, it was the faint dark patch (I'm sure I'm the only one who notices it) that developed on my cheekbone after Gaston's birth that finally induced me to keep that sunscreen right there on my dressing table—and to use it, every day.

If I'm going to be in direct sunlight for an extended period—again, for shooting or for an afternoon by the pool—I cover my face and neck with a complete sun*block*. My dermatologist has given me his

Gaston and I, both well protected from the California sun, play by the pool.

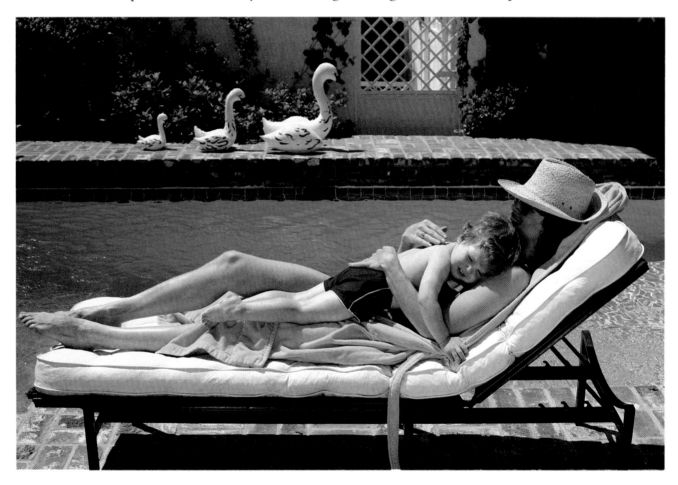

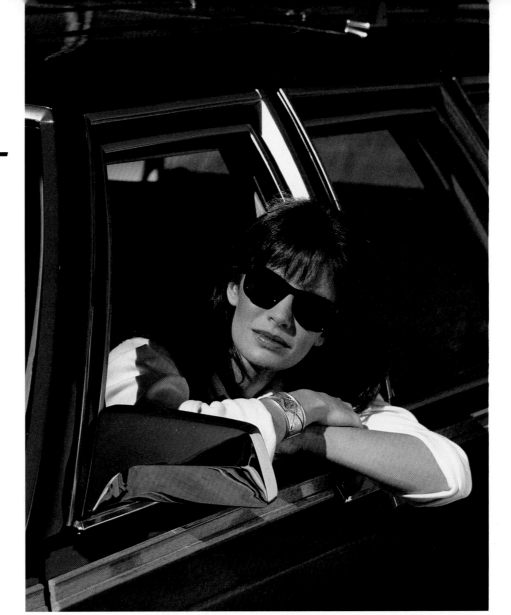

*Sunglasses aren't a movie-
star affectation; they're
wrinkle fighters!*

own formulation, which is clear, so I don't have to walk around with white blobs of cream on my face. But fortunately, even some of the commercial brands are see-through now, especially the total blocks designed for supersensitive areas like the nose, eyes and neck.

Hats and sunglasses come into play when we go, as a family, to the beach or on bicycling adventures. I'm amused by the trend for wearing sunglasses day and night, indoors and out. (That can't be good for your eyes!) But on the other hand, I don't wear them as often as I should. Even for driving I sometimes forget.

It's evident that in the glaring sun, if you're squinting, you should be wearing dark glasses. After all, that squinting is only deepening those lines around your eyes. Besides, sunglasses can be so attractive and even slightly mysterious.

AGING AND SKIN

Everything you read about aging and skin emphasizes the necessity of protection from the sun's harmful rays. What amazes me about so many of the fitness buffs and body-beautiful types, especially visible in Southern California, is that they totally ignore this warning. There they are, as taut and macrobiotically pure as possible, bronzing themselves to a fare-thee-well on the beaches.

I understand how difficult it is as a teenager to take seriously the idea of the cumulative damage blatant sun exposure causes. But when a woman becomes a little more mature, she has to take responsibility for herself, and that includes a decision about sunbathing. I know how attractive a deep tan can make you look, and feel, but I've also seen the long-term effects: leathery chests, accordion-pleated mouths, canyon-deep furrows. Excessive exposure to the sun can also cause certain kinds of cancer and other medical problems. So the choice is up to you.

Sun exposure is, happily, one aging factor that we have control over. Our heredity—the lines that are "mapped" into our faces at birth—is not. So a woman also has to develop some acceptance of lines and wrinkles that *are* going to occur.

I see hints of lines in my own face, but they appear ever so gradually. (Thank goodness, you don't wake up one morning all prunelike and wrinkled! Nature gives you time to adjust to the idea.) The question is: what to do about the lines you don't like?

I haven't yet decided—or had to—about having any injections or plastic surgery. But I assure you, these are options I plan to investigate. In fact, I've already begun my research just by looking around me at women who've had bad surgery (it's sadly obvious) and by talking with friends who'll own up to injections or good surgery.

There's quite a controversy brewing about whether collagen or silicone injections are more effective for filling in tiny lines and wrinkles and plumping up those first, faint creases. I intend to discuss the pros and cons with my dermatologist and other experts in the field before taking any action. So should you.

I do think it's foolish to right out dismiss science's offerings when it comes to bettering our appearance. There do exist low-risk, time-tested methods for ameliorating signs of age. So why not investigate? Believe me, I have no desire to look twenty when I'm forty, but I think every woman wants to look as good as possible. Let's just say I haven't ruled out cosmetic surgery or other techniques if, and when, the time comes. But I might add that I hope never to slip from conscientious concern about my looks into an obsession with age and the changes it brings about in my face. I can't think of an unhappier way to live!

CONVERSATION WITH AN EXPERT: JOLANTA WIBUCH ON SKIN CARE

Jolanta Wibuch is an aesthetician who has for several years run her own very successful skin-care salon in Beverly Hills. After two years of college and several more of training in a dermatological/surgical institute in Krakow, Poland, Jolanta came to the United States and began working at a well-known salon in Chicago. I met her, through the recommendations of friends, when she moved to the Los Angeles branch of Saks Fifth Avenue, where Jolanta ran a franchised skin-care operation before opening her own salon on Wilshire Boulevard. Here, Jolanta and I discuss some of the most-asked skin-related questions that concern every woman, from Jolanta's many famous clients to my own many letter-writing fans.

JS: What's the first thing you do when a new client comes to your salon for help with her skin?

JW: Of course, I first cleanse, then examine her skin, both technically speaking, with the Wood's light and magnifying glass, but also a bit psychologically. With thirty years of experience, I try to determine what's going through this woman's mind about how she looks.

For instance, in talking with her, I can get some sense of how much stress she's under in life. And that can affect the skin's condition tremendously. At the same time, I am typing her skin: dry, normal, oily, or combination. I can certainly tell if she works on having good skin or not.

JS: Do most women know what type of skin they have?

JW: Basically, I think they do. At least, they are not unaware. I think women just like to hear someone else, an authority, confirm what they've already discovered about themselves.

I do find, however, that you have to be very careful about discussing problem skin with a client. I must be very diplomatic; stress the positive aspects; hold out hope.

JS: Do diet and vitamin recommendations come into your program?

JW: No. Not because I'm not convinced diet and possible vitamin deficiencies can't play an enormous role in the status of the skin, but because that is a deep and involved area that is not my field of expertise. I do, however, recommend that my clients consult the experts in these fields when necessary.

JS: Women who never had acne as teenagers write to me that they've developed breakouts and acne in their thirties, even forties. Is this possible?

JW: Certainly. Many women, and men, who never suffered as adolescents find themselves dealing with a sort of acne in their thirties and, for menopausal women, sometimes in their forties, for the first time.

It's a very difficult thing to treat. There are so many factors involved: the stress levels, changes in hormonal levels, activity in the lymph-gland system and nervous system of the individual. My role in serious acne cases is to work with the dermatologist's program of treatment, and most of all, help the client keep his or her skin clean.

One of the biggest problems is, I think, that in trying to dry out the overproductive oil glands, women often actually damage the top layer of their skin with too-harsh soaps and cleansers. I treat acne skin as very, very sensitive skin.

JS: How do you feel about the use of textured scrub mitts or pads for the face? And what about beauty creams with cleansing grains in them?

JW: Well, for the highly sensitive acne skins we were just talking about, I say absolutely not. I think these scrub pads are too rough and can further irritate already fragile skin. That goes for skin that's been overexposed to sun and wind, too. But when you're speaking of more normal skins, I don't mind if a woman wants to use a buffing pad or a product with grains or almond bits in it—anything as long as it's not too rough.

How can she tell? Well, this is something I don't think many experts would say, but I believe women must take some responsibility for their own skins. They have to use their own judgment about whether a product they're using is irritating, and then they have to experiment with using that product less frequently, or not at all.

JS: Is it true that all skins require moisturizer?

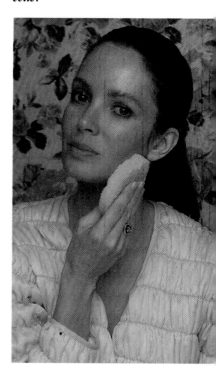

Gentle use of a facial-scrub pad helps exfoliate—that is, rid skin of dead surface cells.

JW: Well, yes, in the sense that even oily skins often have dry patches. And the classic combination skin is dry on the cheeks and forehead, and oily down through the nose and chin.

An extremely lightweight moisturizer might be called for on even slightly oily sections, while the drier parts of the face, of course, require richer creams. It's just a question of dealing with your skin realistically, not as if it's one, consistent entity.

JS: You do steam cleaning during your salon facials. Do you recommend this practice for everyone?

JW: Basically, yes. If I see some broken capillaries around the nose, for instance, I would cover them before steaming—and always cover the eye area. And it must be a gentle steaming, not too hot or too close to the skin, or you can do damage.

JS: Some women write that they use eye creams at night, only to awaken with unusually puffy eyes in the morning. Is this a common problem?

JW: The eye area is so fragile and needing of care that I believe in eye creams, absolutely. I think when women have this problem of puffiness, it's because they used too rich or too much cream. Or they've chosen a product with preservatives or fragrance in it that might cause a reaction like that.

Even the thirsty skin around the eyes can only absorb so much moisture, so I advise patting an eye cream on, gently, with a fingertip, and then ten to fifteen minutes later—or before you go to bed, anyway—removing the excess with a tissue or cotton.

By the way, as you already know, I always tell my clients to buy the surgical cotton that comes in one long roll rather than preformed cotton balls. I believe it's gentler, and it's often cheaper, than these so-called "cosmetic" cotton balls.

JS: There seem to be so many different types of facial masks available—cleansing masks, pore-tightening masks, moisturizing masks. Which ones do you feel are effective for which skin types?

JW: First of all, I only believe in masks as effective for a moisturizing function. And for that reason, I recommend them for any but the oiliest skins. Commercially available products, or even masks you make at home out of avocado or egg yolks, can be very nourishing

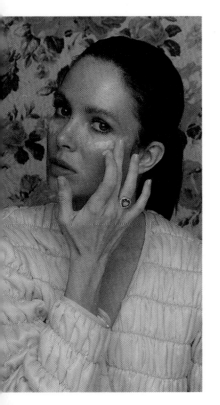

Delicate skin around the eye deserves the special attention of a specifically formulated moisturizer.

for dry and normal skins. I tell women to think of a once-a-week mask as an investment in their skin.

JS: Do you think drinking alcohol has a necessarily adverse effect on the skin?

JW: Not necessarily. Some women—and they don't have to be alcoholics—do have a bad reaction: redness in the face, broken veins or capillaries around the nose. When I see what I suspect are these reactions to alcohol, I normally recommend, diplomatically, that the client visit a dermatologist, if she's concerned about the reddening of her skin.

JS: As a nonsmoker, I'm very curious if you can tell by looking at her skin if a woman smokes cigarettes.

JW: I will not say that I can detect from her skin's condition whether or not a client smokes. I think smoking's negative effects are more subtle, more indirect than that. It's a question of oxygenation and blood circulation. If anything, I can tell a smoker by her voice more than by her complexion.

JS: There seems to be a controversy developing about jogging, whether it makes women look older, or better.

JW: Of course, a lot of my clients are joggers, and I wouldn't want to discourage them from that, from getting out and exercising. But I sometimes attempt discreetly to steer them toward less vigorous exercise like walking or hiking, because I've noticed that many joggers seem to be straining as they run along, frowning and glaring with the effort.

If you do run, I believe it should be at a pace you can handle and one which doesn't create a strain that's bound to show up in the face, as wrinkles, sooner or later. Also, correctly fitted running shoes and running on a soft surface are very important. Pounding away on asphalt or cement can't be helpful for the elastic elements in your skin.

JS: Are you an advocate of doing regular facial exercises?

JW: Facial exercises are a very interesting topic. I do believe they can be beneficial, but there's a problem. The muscles in the face have to be dealt with very carefully, so carefully that I would never recommend a woman attempt facial exercises on her own, without an expert right by her side to see that she's doing them correctly. Because that's pretty impractical for most women, and because I feel so strongly that facial exercises are difficult to do right, I suppose I'd have to say "skip them."

JS: You and I both live in California. And I know you're a sportswoman who likes skiing and sailing. Yet every skin expert warns about the damaging effects of the sun. What's realistic?

JW: First, I must comment on the fact that I find the sun here much stronger than sun in Europe. But, regardless of that—or because of it —I'm serious when I say that a woman should not walk out of her house without some sort of sun protection. Obviously, blue-eyed, fair-skinned women are most susceptible to damage. But even olive- and dark-skinned women must wear some protection. Fortunately, today there are many moisturizers and foundations that already have PABA or some other blocking or screening ingredient in them.

I'm pained when I'm at the beach or skiing and see very young girls, wearing no protection, who've already burned their faces. The difficult thing is that they won't see the negative effects for years to come.

JS: What's the best way to find a skin-care specialist? Should you listen to friends? Is it fair to judge her potential performance by the condition of her skin?

JW: Yes, I think recommendations from friends are very useful. But you have to see if you develop a rapport with that aesthetician. If for some reason you feel you'll never really develop trust in her or her advice, it's a waste of time.

As far as judging her expertise by the condition of her skin, I think that's a little unfair. I'll tell you why. I'm convinced that a large part of your skin's condition is attributable to your heredity, to your parents. Therefore, you can't really change an extremely oily skin. You can only keep it as clean and blemish-free as possible, with constant work. You cannot change a sensitive skin, only treat it gently and try not to irritate it.

The point is that an aesthetician may not have been born with perfect skin. And she must work on it to make it look and feel as good as possible. But none of that means she isn't totally qualified to do the same for you—make your skin look and feel its best.

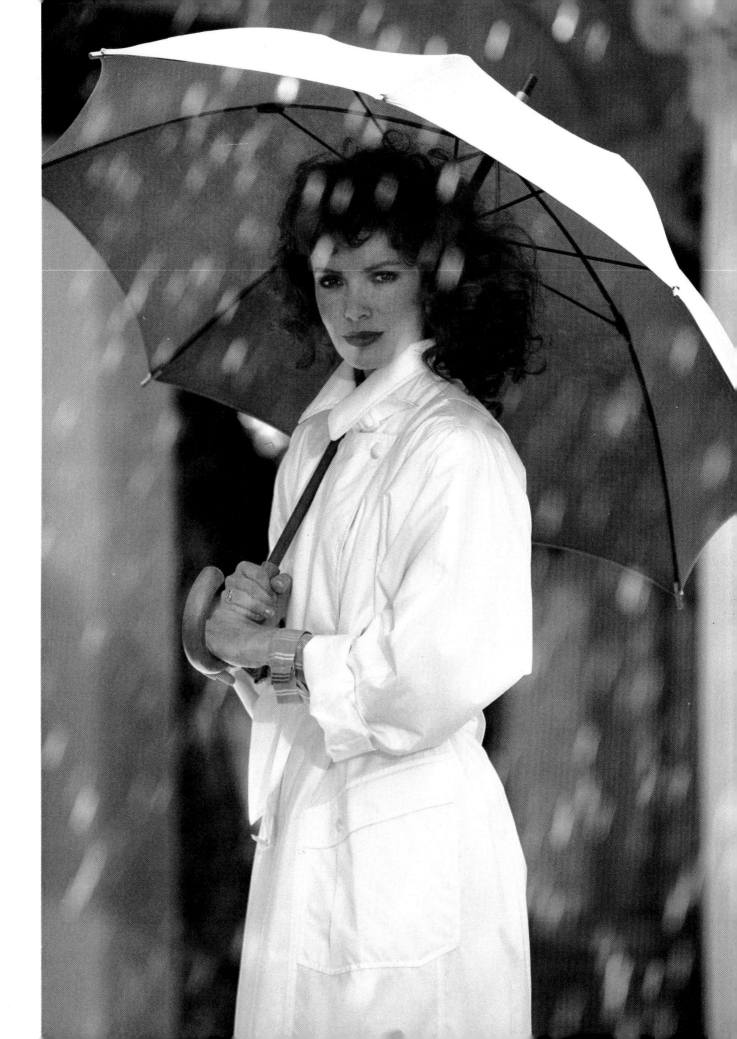

JS: I think every woman over the age of twenty-five wants to know what a facialist can do about wrinkles, before and after they appear.

JW: Again, wrinkles are, to some extent, genetically mapped into your face, scheduled to appear at a certain age. But I also believe that we help cause our own wrinkles by our attitude toward life, and carelessness about sun and pollution exposure.

Aside from always using sunblock—and a visor or hat when you're playing sports like tennis—there are a couple of things you can do. For instance, I sometimes ask a client to watch herself in the mirror while she talks on the telephone. She often discovers facial expressions and tics that aren't particularly appealing or necessary: biting a lip, knitting her brows. Becoming aware of these useless facial movements—I'm not talking about smile lines, now—can help you stop making them.

You can even practice a technique of isolation, on the forehead, for example. Start by sitting quietly, with your eyes closed, and just concentrate on relaxing those muscles in your forehead. Try to isolate them and let them go. Then, again in front of a mirror while you're on the phone, try to keep this area relaxed, even as you talk. Mastering this exercise could save you at least a few of those deep forehead lines in later years.

Another way women participate in their own wrinkles develops, oddly enough, out of vanity. I do meet women who, as they age, experience a change in their eyesight. Yet they're too vain to get glasses. It's ridiculous. If you can't see, you squint. If you squint, you create unnecessary wrinkles.

Sunglasses are a must, too. But fortunately, in California anyway, *everyone* seems happy to wear sunglasses—all the time!

In America, aestheticians are not involved, but dermatologists do have their own techniques for wrinkle removal. Dermabrasion—peeling away a layer of the skin, either mechanically or chemically—is one approach. Lines can be filled in or plumped up with minuscule injections of silicone or collagen, too. If a woman is considering any of these options, she should, of course, consult a qualified dermatologist.

JS: I think some women are intimidated when they first go for a professional facial. What is your advice?

JW: Well, the most important thing is for the woman to remember that she doesn't have to do anything she doesn't want to do. Most reputable skin-care specialists will happily explain each step of the facial being given, and why it's deemed necessary. But the client is free to say no to any step she's unsure of.

I'm thinking primarily of the machines used in many salons. I don't believe they're terribly useful. In fact, some of them are potentially dangerous in untrained or unskilled hands. A woman simply shouldn't allow herself to be talked into their use on *her* face!

JS: Do you have any way of permanently removing freckles or age spots?

JW: Women do come to me with unwanted freckles or discolorations caused by anything from sun exposure to the birth-control pill to age. I can diminish them, temporarily, with bleaching creams. But unless the discoloration fades on its own—as it often does with the birth-control pills or in pregnancy-related cases—the lightening effects are temporary because brown freckles and spots are the sites of pigmentation in the skin cells themselves.

Bleaching creams are particularly useful during the winter months, but when spring comes, and you go back out into an increasingly strong sun, those brown patches are very likely to reappear.

JS: Surely some of your clients must have had plastic surgery—either just on their eyes or a full face-lift. How does the approach to skin care change after such surgery?

JW: The step-by-step regimen doesn't change that much because the skin isn't changed as to type. Oily skin is still oily; dry is still dry. What is critical is to be particularly careful about the manipulation of the skin, because its elasticity is usually diminished after surgery.

I'm very careful about doing facial massages on such clients, and advise them to be extremely gentle when applying and removing skin-care products and makeup at home. And women who've had surgery have to be fiercely careful about exposure to the sun, but then, I believe every woman should.

JS: Can a woman do effective facial massage on herself?

JW: Yes, if she learns from a pro. Sometimes, at my salon, I see women beating at their necks or on their cheeks, thinking they're doing some good. They're not. But especially while applying creams and things, with competent instruction, a woman can learn to make it a very pleasurable experience. There's truth in the notion that up-

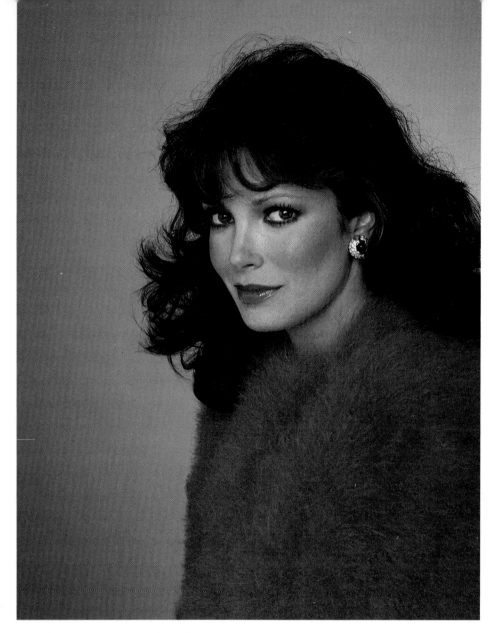

ward sweeps are preferable when applying or removing any product from the face.

To some women, I teach easy pressure-point massage. That way, there's no danger of overmanipulation of tender skin. Plus, it feels great!

JS: With all your experience, what are the areas of at-home skin care where most women go wrong?

JW: My answers are both sort of attitudinal. First, women have to realize that even if they go to a skin-care specialist regularly, *they* have to do the work, day-in and day-out. How many times does a woman go out and buy a whole new skin-care regimen, use it religiously for three or four nights, and then forget about it? You have to make good skin care a habit, just like brushing your teeth. It's your skin, and it's your discipline that will ultimately determine how good it looks.

Second, many women forget that skin care means you have to take care of the face *and* the neck and chest, *and* the hands. Necks are so often neglected, and they need the same moisturizing and sunscreening treatment your face does. As for your hands, lack of moisturizer and sunblock shows up there often before anywhere else. That's why they say hands give away your true age. One of the best things you can do for yourself, starting now, is to vow never to expose your hands to the sun again, certainly not without a strong sunblock cream on them.

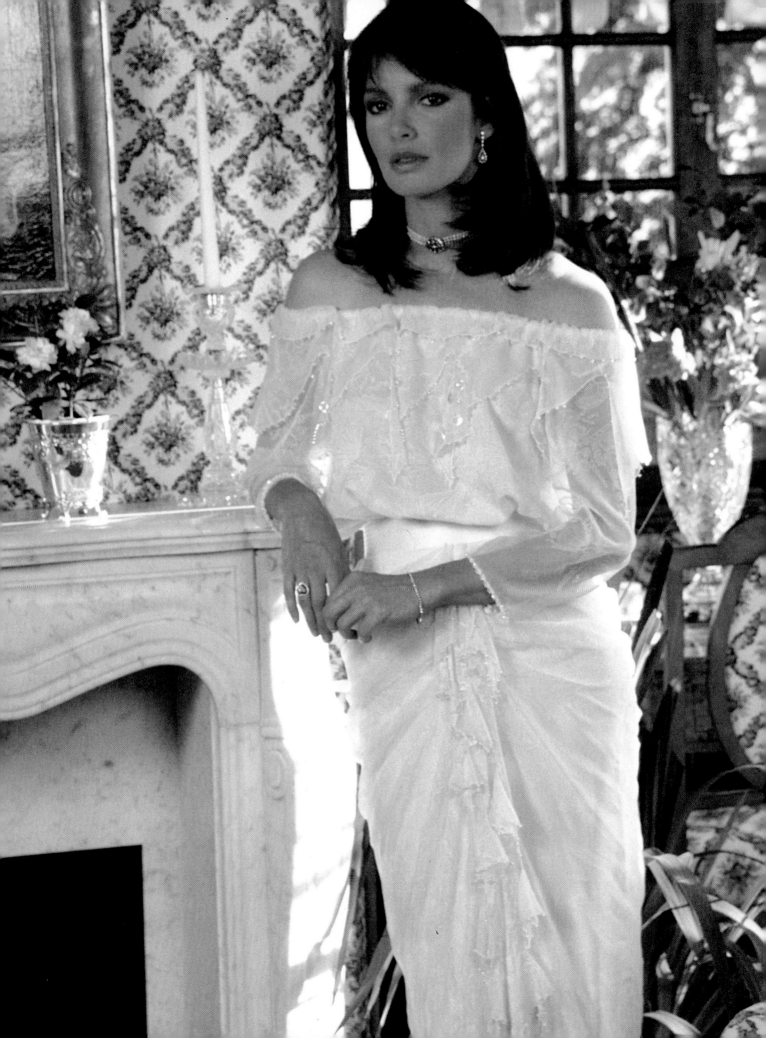

CHAPTER 5

Gentle Hands and Perfect Feet

I've always felt that elegant, graceful hands are a wonderfully feminine attribute. I don't necessarily mean pampered hands that really do nothing—just ones that look that way. After all, what could better inspire a man to slip a little diamond bauble on your finger? And when you're a mother of small children, the importance of having soft, gentle hands becomes all the more obvious.

Your nails are no less important. And while nothing can spoil a well-coiffed, beautifully dressed woman's look faster than ragged, unkempt nails, I'm not a big fan of clawlike, blood-red nails, either. As a teenager, I experimented with all different shapes and colors before I settled on *my* look: healthy, softly rounded nails, polished in a natural-look color, to elongate my smooth hands.

I'll admit that one reason I've come to favor subtler nail lacquers for most-of-the-time wear is that with work, raising Gaston, and just living my life, it's a lot easier not to have to worry about last-minute disasters of chipped polish. If a pale, pale peach color or transparent pink starts to wear off or takes a beating, I can let it go until I have the time for a complete manicure. Also, I truly prefer the cleanliness of the look.

There's no question that when you do choose a stronger nail-lacquer shade—as I do for photography sessions or important evenings—matching it to your lipstick or your dress is a bit old-fashioned. Not wrong, just needlessly limiting. In general, I think your fingertips ought to be dressed in a tone slightly darker than your lipstick, and simply not clash with your clothing.

SMOOTH HANDS

Keeping hands soft and silky is not an easy feat for today's superactive woman. For starters, I keep a good hand moisturizer next to the sink in my bathroom, in the kitchen and in my son's bathroom so that I can smooth it on every time I wash my hands. A mini-tube tucked into your purse isn't a bad idea, either.

Going to bed with plastic or cotton gloves over richly moisturized hands is a good idea, too, but it may be a little tricky if there's a man sharing that bed with you. What does make sense is to select a time when you'll be wearing gloves anyway—housework, gardening—and then schedule your at-least-once-a-week deep-moisturizing treatment. No one need know!

When you go for a professional facial or massage (both experiences I highly recommend) you'll often find your hands coated with a rich cream and then slipped into warming mitts, which are sort of like electric blankets for your hands. The heat helps make the emollients

Busy hands require real protection: gloves, sunscreen and moisturizer.

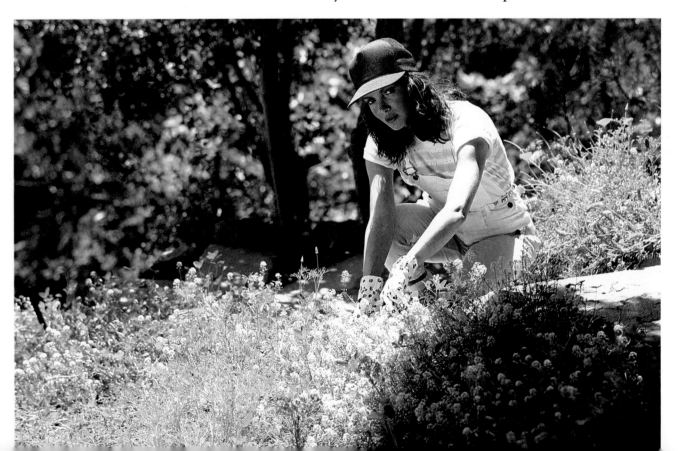

in the cream penetrate better and faster. You can replicate the effect by using plastic gloves—the kind doctors wear or those included with home hair-coloring kits—for your secret hand-softening sessions.

It's so often said that it must be true: hands are the first thing to give away a woman's age. So I make taking care of mine an automatic ritual. That means wearing gloves as often as possible when I do housework, the gardening and even when I drive. They are essential, too, when I play sports to avoid calluses and blisters. I also wear them outside in cold weather, of course. In sunny weather, my hands deserve sunblock, frequently replenished, as much as my face does.

I don't hesitate to use facial-quality masks and sloughing creams on my hands, either. Again, the theory being if it's good enough for my face . . .

Fortunately I don't have to deal with them yet, but telltale age spots, I'm told, can often be diminished with one of those bleaching creams available in department and specialty stores.

A PERFECT TEN

If you've never been too good at giving yourself a manicure, or if you just want to brush up on your skills, I recommend going for a first-rate professional job. Just once, and if you really pay attention, you'll have the techniques down. It may be an extravagance, but I have a weekly appointment with a professional manicurist who comes to my home. But if you can't swing a regular weekly appointment, it's always good to have confidence that you can do it yourself.

A professional manicure is a great treat and a learning experience.

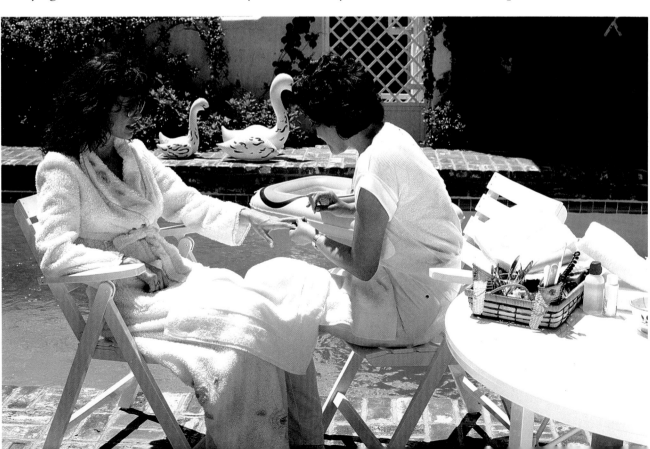

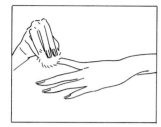

1. Remove all traccs of polish with a nongreasy remover, with cotton or tissue.

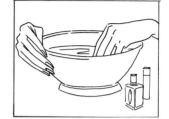

2. Soak nails in warm, sudsy water or a hot-oil nail treatment.

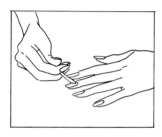

3. Dry hands; push back cuticles and clean behind nail edges with orangewood stick wrapped in cotton.

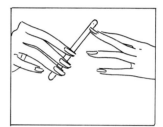

4. File nails to rounded shape the width of your fingertip; no metal files. Ideally, they'll be about one-half inch long.

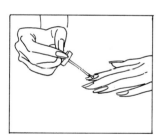

5. Apply ridge-filler if needed; then base coat.

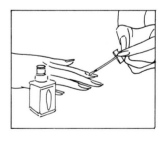

6. Let dry before adding one or two coats of colored nail lacquer.

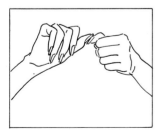

7. Test dryness by lightly touching one polished nail surface against another; if they stick, wait.

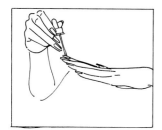

8. Apply top coat or sealer; allow to dry thoroughly.

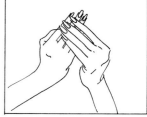

9. Special tip: when polish is completely dry, apply hand cream. Then peel off any excess polish that's gotten on your skin.

Remember your toenails deserve the same careful treatment as your fingernails.

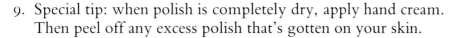

You'll notice, first of all, that the pro has all her tools assembled: a fresh white towel; a good light; a bowl of warm, sudsy water or even a warmed-oil treatment; cuticle scissors, an emery board, an orange-wood stick, and, of course, remover, cotton balls and polish.

As any leftover polish is removed, the professional manicurist will examine your nails for strength and length. Though I'm a firm believer in a good diet's contribution to both hair and nails, heredity also plays a big role in how healthy your fingernails are. But no matter what your genes, keeping your nails manicured and polished is a positive step toward the prettiest hands possible.

That's not to say that some difficulties can't be overcome with one of several false-nail techniques. Wrapping, for example, is the application of tissue-thin bits of cotton or silk "paper" to strengthen splits. Medium-to-dark polish is a necessary follow-up to these mending methods.

I'm not crazy about the myriad porcelain-powder-and-liquid-glue nail-builders available under countless do-it-yourself brand names. But since they do allow your own nails to grow out underneath, I prefer them to techniques that require the roughening of your real nails so that tips can be attached. Whole, glue-on nails that you simply trim to fit over the existing ones should, I think, be saved for true eleventh-hour disasters. I've found they just don't work very successfully beyond a night's wear, and the sensation of touch with these false nails is a bit distorted and awkward.

The manicurist's second step is to soak your nails in the softening solution—meant really to soften your cuticles more than the nails themselves. Having dried your hand on her towel, she'll then gently cut away any ragged skin or excess cuticle (not advised at home unless you're particularly adept) and push the cuticles back, ever so gently, with the flattened end of the orangewood stick swathed in cotton. The same stick's pointed end, again wrapped in a wisp of cotton, is used to clean behind the nails.

Filing comes next, and this is, I think, where many women go wrong. There are fads in fingernail shape just as in anything else concerning feminine beauty. Remember the long, squared-off nails of the '60s? And look at today's pointy, punk-rock nails. But the fact is, short to medium-length nails (that means nails extending one-quarter inch to one-half inch beyond the end of your finger), gently rounded to match the width of your finger itself, look best.

They're also the healthiest. You weaken nails if you file them to a width narrower than your fingers. They're liable to split and break at the sides. Also, there's a harmony of line when the nails aren't decidedly narrower than the fingers. Think of it this way: you'd never wear a ring that was too small for your finger, would you? Don't try to create too-small nails. It throws the proportions off.

Experts will tell you that you must always file in one direction. That's great advice if you're more skilled than I with an emery board. (You weren't even thinking about using a *metal* nail file, were you?) But if I work in a relaxed fashion—not like a convict trying to saw his way out of jail—on dry, clean nails and concentrate on filing at a right angle to the nail edge, things work out pretty well. The goal is to achieve a smooth, even edge in an attractive arc.

Needless to say, if one or several nails are dramatically longer than the others, the professional will undoubtedly suggest that you simply cut down those errant nails, rather than build up all the others.

Next comes ridge-filler and/or base coat. This step is tempting to skip if you're doing the work yourself, but it's important—like preparing a canvas before painting—and it really contributes to long-wearing, glossy color. Slight irregularities are normal in nails and can be covered over. Deep ridges and malformations can be signs of some nutritional deficiency or other condition and should be brought to the attention of your doctor.

For some reason, I prefer doing my right hand first. I suppose it's because I'm right-handed and feel surer of not messing up the wet nails on my right hand while I attend to my left. Base coat, like all nail products, is applied from the cuticle up to the tip, in even, flowing strokes. Usually, the time it takes to do the other hand will allow the first five nails to dry sufficiently.

As you'll learn from watching the pro, the actual nail color is applied the same way, from cuticle to tip, in light strokes. For a really finished effect, the undersides of the nail tips are colored, too. Depending on the depth of the shade you've chosen and the coverage desired, you'll want to apply one or two full coats—with three to five minutes between for drying.

I've mentioned that I prefer a see-through appearance for my own nails. This look can be created with what is called a French manicure. An old-fashioned approach that's returning to vogue, the French manicure precedes the base-coat step with a clear, white polish that's artfully painted on, just over the naturally white part of the nail tip. After that come the base coat and a pale, transparent color of polish.

If your nails are particularly fragile, it's silly not to take advantage of all the fabulous fashion colors that now come in nail-hardening formulations, some with fibers, some without.

Finally, a clear liquid-sealer coat goes on, to protect the polish and heighten the shine. Sealer can be applied under the tips, too.

The hardest part, for me, anyway, is waiting till my nails are completely dry. If you get fidgety, you might want to try one of those quick-dry sprays or top coats. At home, and as they do in some salons, you can speed up the drying process by plunging your nails into ice-cold water. Just be careful when drying your hands!

Do not do anything that jeopardizes your perfect manicure, including fishing in your purse for keys or trying to "slip" your hands through your coat sleeves. There's nothing more dismaying than smudging still-wet polish.

An expert manicurist knows how to test just-polished nails by touching them with her fingertip. Don't try it yourself. What you can do is bring two nails together, one from each hand, of course, with the lightest contact possible. If they stick even slightly, they're not yet completely dry.

Another trick I've learned for doing my own nails: if you've been a bit sloppy and gotten polish on the skin surrounding the nail, don't worry. And don't try to remove it while the polish is still wet. Wait till everything's completely dry, apply hand cream and then just peel off the polish. You'll see; it comes off readily.

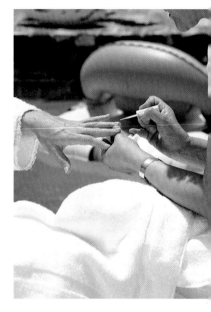

Medium-length nails, lacquered in a pale color, are easier to maintain.

FEMININE FEET

My feet—you're probably thinking—why, they're the last thing I need, or have the time, to worry about! I used to feel much the same way. But every time I slip my feet into a revealing pair of high-heeled sandals on a fashion photography shoot or simply take off my espadrilles at the pool, I realize how important attractive feet can be.

Also, years of dance training have made me aware that taking care of my feet means they're much less likely to hurt. We've all been there at that party where you look terrific, but your feet are killing you. In two words: no fun. And it's usually because you haven't been giving your feet the attention they deserve.

The professional pedicure is also an extravagance. But the fact is, if you can steal a few extra minutes after your bath, just once a week, you can keep your own feet smooth and well manicured.

Before we go on to the step-by-step procedure, let me share one little thing I've learned about going to a salon. If I'm pressed for time, I always have the pro do everything *but* apply the polish. I've found that even if I double up and have a manicure and pedicure simultaneously, somehow my toenails end up sticking to my stockings, often hours later. My trick is to apply the polish myself, at home, so I can walk around barefoot, with those charming cotton wads between my toes, for as long as it takes for the polish to dry thoroughly to a hard, glossy finish.

GETTING DOWN TO IT

Feet mustn't be neglected either, especially during summer or warm-climate getaways.

Bathtime is the best time for your weekly at-home pedicure, because the warm, soapy water of the tub ensures that your feet and toenails will be clean and soft. The process will actually begin *in* the bath, as that's where you use a pumice stone or sloughing cream to work off

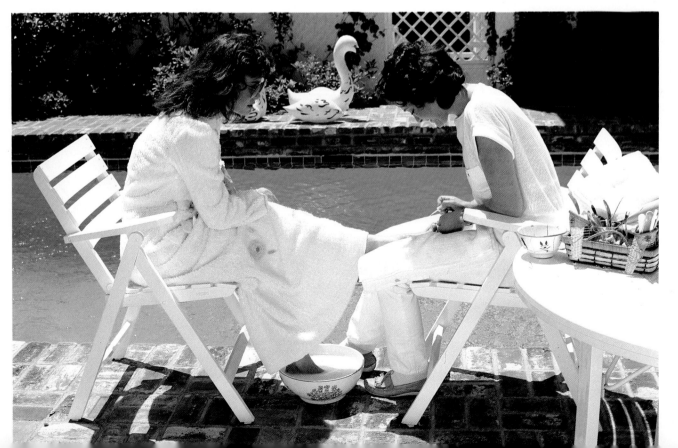

callused, rough skin around the heels, along the sides of the soles and on the balls of the feet. Even if pumicing does tickle the bottoms of your feet unmercifully, the results are worth it. Corns and warts, however, should be left to a podiatrist to handle.

When you're out of the bath and toweled dry, don't neglect your feet when you apply your body lotion. Then wrap yourself up in a favorite robe and find someplace comfortable, with a good, direct light nearby. You'll need to have gathered polish remover, cuticle cream, an orangewood stick, nail scissors, an emery board, a towel and some cotton, or one of those cute little wavy rubber wedges made specifically for separating your toes while polish can dry.

After the removal of any residual polish, the application of a softening cuticle cream is a good place to start your pedicure. Massage it into the rough skin all around the toenails and into the cuticles themselves, of course. Then use the orangewood stick, always gently, to push back the cuticle. I don't believe in cutting them unless there's a part that's drastically ragged. Metal cuticle clippers are the only tool to use, in this case.

Do use scissors—they seem less brutal than nail clippers—to trim overlong nails, and follow with the orangewood stick to clean behind the nail. What you don't want is long toenails! They should end where your toes end.

The emery board comes next, to shape and smooth the just-cut nail edges. Shaping isn't a big issue here, since there's to be no nail extending beyond the edge of the toe. However, you'll want to pay particular attention to the corners of the nails. For toes only, the nails *should* be filed inward a bit, rounded, really, to avoid the aggravation of ingrown toenails.

You can use rubber wedges, wads of cotton, or even carefully folded tissues to separate the toes before you begin with the base coat. Yes, your toes do get the full treatment your fingernails get. To avoid disappointing smudges during application, proceed big toe to little on your right foot and little toe to big on your left foot if you're right-handed. For left-handed women, of course, the reverse is easiest.

Base coat/ridge-filler is followed by one or two coats of colored polish. And though I'm pretty conservative about fingernail-polish colors, I'm a touch more daring when it comes to my toes: bright reds, real corals, pretty pinks are all great.

Of course, if this pedicure precedes a big evening out when you're going to be wearing open-toed shoes, do take into consideration a lacquer shade that won't clash with your shoes. The shade need not match the color of your shoes—green toenails?—or your dress or

*Tennis shoes make great
sense for active feet.*

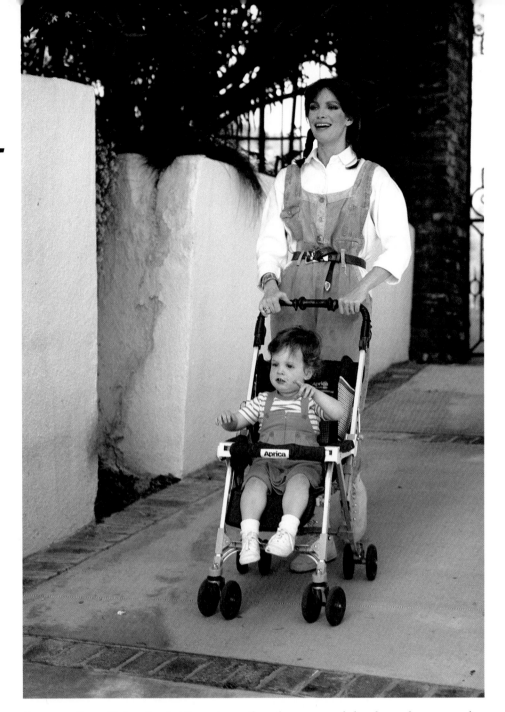

fingernail polish. And if you prefer the natural look, whatever the occasion, you can skip polish altogether and simply use a professional buffer to bring toenails to a healthy shine and glow.

Colored nail lacquer is, as you know, topped by a sealer/top coat once it's dry. Then comes the allover drying time, at least a half hour. If you're at home, that's no problem. You can just pad around bare-foot with cotton between your toes and not mess up your handiwork.

FOOT NOTES

Doctors have told me again and again that American women can be positively masochistic when it comes to their feet. The point I'm making is don't let vanity talk you into shoes that are too small or heels that are too high. And that applies to everything from the perfect little evening pump to running shoes. Wearing poorly fitted shoes can cause trouble, ranging from annoying, recurring blisters to really quite serious malformations.

Also, knowing full well how terrific high heels can make a woman's legs look, I'm also aware of how off-balance and tired they can make you. I still wear them sometimes, of course. But I switch to flats or tennis shoes whenever possible, especially now that there's a three-year-old in my life. After all, you really can't move very fast on those stilts!

Wearing clean socks or stockings is also important for healthy feet. They're often the only thing between you and blisters. If you wear knee-highs make sure they're not too tight or constricting at the calf.

When I'm wearing sandals or really casual beach shoes that don't call for stockings or socks, I smooth talcum powder all over my feet and the insides of my shoes to keep from developing "hot spots"—you know, that uncomfortable burning sensation at the heels or the balls of the feet.

Going barefoot is one of the great joys of beach life, and I take advantage of every opportunity. Not only does it feel deliciously free, there's a beauty bonus. Walking on the sand is quite good exercise for your foot and calf muscles.

When I'm indoors, it's a simple flat or ballet slipper. On the street, you really need something more constructed, with a sole that'll give you support so you won't constantly feel you're literally pounding the pavement.

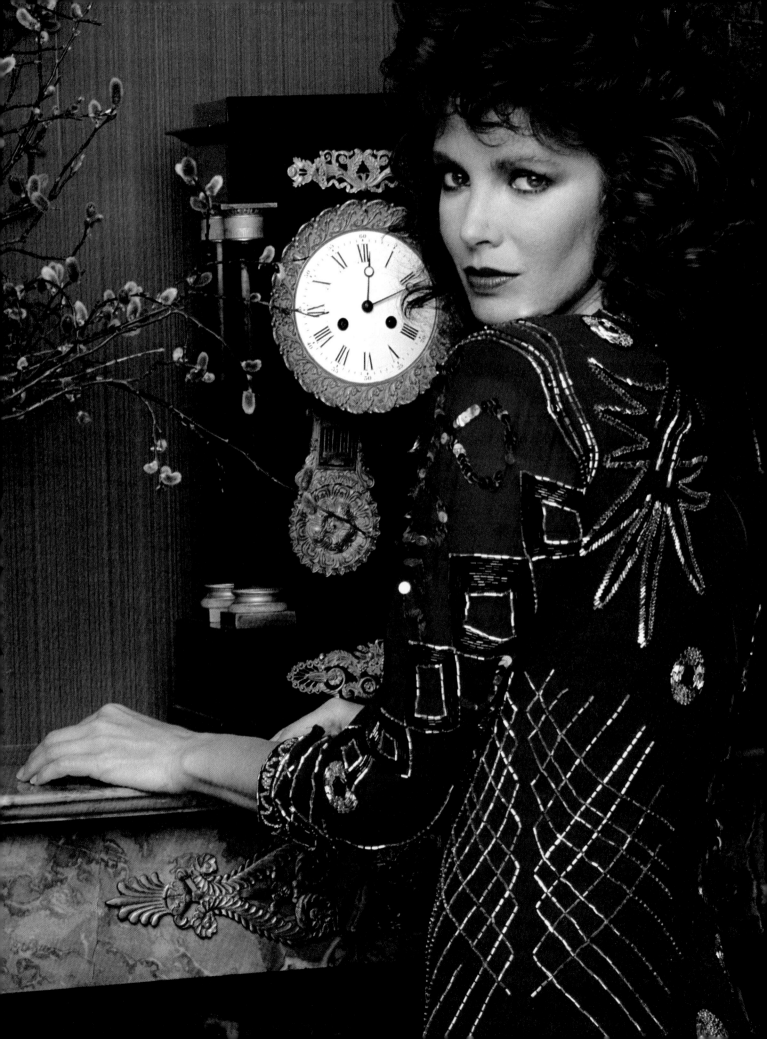

A Fabulous Face

I probably inherited my preference for the natural look from my mother. She never did, and still doesn't, wear much makeup. And neither did I until I began performing in school dramatics and then studying dance and modeling professionally. It was only then that I gained a real appreciation for how makeup can enhance your looks when properly applied—emphasis on *properly applied*.

I still marvel at the various looks that can be coaxed out of one face —mine—depending on the requirements of the role or the job at hand. When I played Jacqueline Bouvier Kennedy, for example, it was the thicker, darker, drawn-on eyebrows that made so much difference in creating a likeness.

For Sally Fairfax, my character in "George Washington," we were very faithful to the notions of makeup during the eighteenth century. Well-brought-up women of that era could pinch a little color into their lips and cheeks, but wearing lipstick and especially rouge was considered "fast." The natural look in those days really was natural.

Today, a woman can use a vast array of cosmetics without ruining her reputation. But many women, myself included, still prefer that natural look, and we use makeup to achieve it. That sounds contradictory, I know. But even when I played the glamorous Kelly Garrett, or when I do commercials or still photographs for Max Factor, there are no great exaggerations in my appearance. I certainly wear more makeup than I would ordinarily, but underneath it's still me.

It's on fashion-magazine sittings that I can really sit back and let a makeup artist and hairdresser go. I get the fun of experimenting, without having to do the work! I usually let them have pretty free rein, partially because I realize it's their job to give me a new look, *their* look. But I never go in front of a camera when I'm not pleased with my appearance; I just can't perform well for a photographer or director under those circumstances.

I've learned an enormous amount from all the extraordinary artists who have done my makeup for films, TV and print. But at home, spending hours in front of a makeup mirror just isn't my thing. Precisely because film makeup, when *I* do my own eyes, can take forty-five minutes and still photography can demand an hour or more, I've picked up the simplest techniques possible to achieve a look that's right for my real life, that pleases my husband and me, and that I can accomplish in about ten to fifteen minutes in the morning, or in no more than thirty minutes before going out at night.

If I do spend an hour getting ready, that's makeup *and* hair—and Gaston is usually in the bathroom with me, so much of the time is actually playtime.

BE PREPARED

When I'm at home doing my own makeup, I always do it at the bathroom sink where water is available, the lighting is good and all my equipment is organized in sliding compartments under the sink. I have a high stool there, though I most often do my makeup standing up.

I first secure my hair away from my face with giant aluminum hairdresser's clips, called Yoyettes, before thoroughly cleansing my face, with either a dry-skin soap or a liquid cleanser and water. Then I apply a mild astringent, and if there's a little breakout or spot, a touch of clear, prescription medicine. I next smooth on a lightweight moisturizer and an eye cream and, if I'm going to be outside, a clear-but-total sunblock.

After this preparation process, I leave my face alone for five to seven

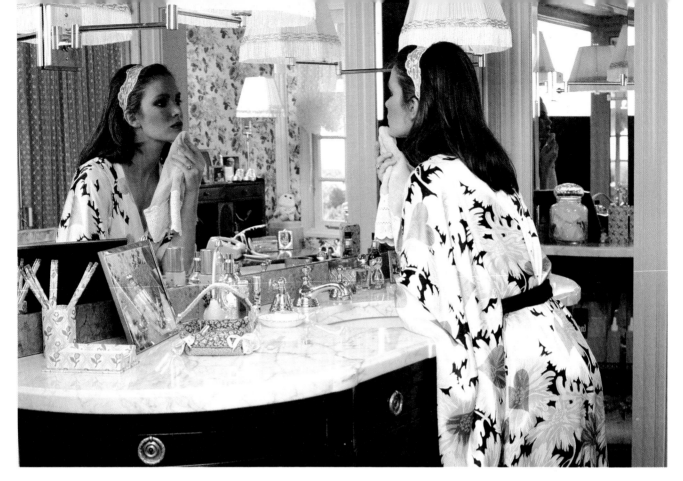

minutes, mostly to absorb all the moisture in the skin-care products. If you apply color immediately, you often get uneven lay-down; that is, the moisturizer can sort of "grab" on to the color in certain spots, making it look splotchy.

Preparing your skin—cleansing and moisturizing—is the essential first step in putting on makeup.

LAYING A FOUNDATION

A light hand is my motto when it comes to applying makeup. And nothing is more important than clean, healthy skin. All the makeup in the world isn't going to make you look your best if you've ignored the good skin care we talked about in chapter 4.

The very first thing you have to consider is your skin's tone. Most women have skin that is not an even, pure color; it might have a reddish or a yellowish cast to it. Color correctors, prefoundation lotions that are tinted green or mauve, are the answer, respectively, to that problem. For further evening of tone, you must then choose a foundation that coordinates with your natural, or color-corrected, tone. Don't attempt to *change* your skin's color with a foundation makeup.

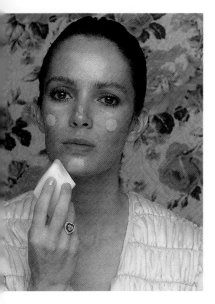

Always use a makeup sponge to blend foundation to an even finish.

A special primer on the eyelids helps color stay on and stay true.

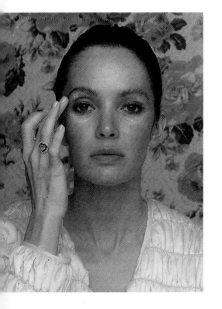

Since I must wear foundation for my work, I sometimes skip it when I'm on my own time. If you feel naked without it, and wear foundation daily, be certain to wash it off completely every night before bed. Your skin has to be allowed a rest, too!

I'm always a bit dismayed when I see women in department stores or wherever, testing a foundation product on their wrists or the back of their hands. You're not going to wear it there, so it doesn't make much sense to color-compare that way, does it? Yes, right there in the cosmetics department, you should dot a little on your face and blend it to determine if the color's right for you. (Don't wear foundation if you're shopping for a new one.)

Having said that you shouldn't try to alter your skin tone with foundation, I might add that you can get away with going a shade or two darker or lighter, in a transitional season, when your tan's fading, for example.

I've found that most professional makeup artists use a makeup sponge for foundation application. They all agree it goes on better, more evenly that way. Though I've been known to dab it on and spread it with my fingertips, I'm finally convinced. Now I keep a fresh supply of those wedge-shaped makeup sponges on hand, always.

For my combination skin, I use a water-based foundation (as opposed to oil-based ones that are better for drier skins). Even so, I always dilute it with more water—a one-to-one ratio of Evian or California tap water—for ultrasheer coverage.

I own several shades of foundation and use them according to the time of year, and how much color I have, or am going to have, in my face. Each, I might add, contains some degree of sunblock, too.

I dot on dime-sized blobs—a couple on my forehead, one on each cheek, one each for the nose and chin—and blend them with the sponge, all the way down, including my neck.

When you don't want a full foundation makeup, I've discovered that you *can* just blend a little foundation, carefully, into off-color areas such as around the nose or under the eyes.

THE EYES HAVE IT

Eye makeup really is fun in the different effects you can achieve and the changes you can make. I insist my eyes are green, though they do tend to look blue or gray in photos, depending on what I'm wearing, or what color my eye shadow is. In any case, eye makeup for me begins with a special primer, Max Factor's Professional Eyeshadow Base, that I dot on my lids and blend with a fingertip to help my eye color stay on and stay true.

In the area around but not under the eye, on either side of the bridge of my nose, and sometimes at its base, I apply and blend a flesh-toned concealer stick. I use a shade of concealer that's just a bit lighter than my foundation—brightening these in-the-shadows areas is the point, after all—but it's nowhere near white.

White concealers and foundations are a real mistake, I think, because white makes things leap forward to the eye. When you're concealing, or highlighting a brow, for that matter, you don't want the affected area to be the first thing an observer sees but rather the thing he or she doesn't notice at all.

When I first started wearing serious makeup, I wore more than I do now, and blue eye shadow was *it* for me. Just blue. Today I'm much more likely to choose a subtler, more sophisticated shade of slate, charcoal, mocha brown, or plum, in a powder shadow that I can put on with a sponge applicator or easy-to-control pencil. The new powder pencils now available are the best of both worlds, and seem designed with people like me in mind.

I line my eyes just along the lash line, top and bottom, and then smudge the color with a sponge-tipped stick or my finger, so that no clear *line* shows. In my experience, it seems that brown liner can make blue eyes look bluer, green eyes greener. So, clearly, matching eye shadow to eye color isn't necessary.

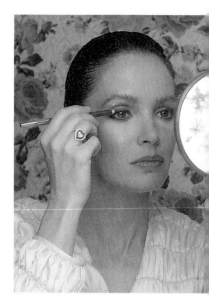

Liner goes on just along the lashes.

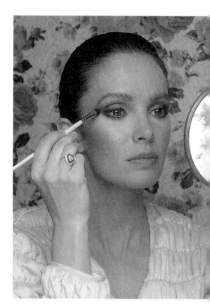

Apply powder shadow after liner.

Use an eyelash curler to give eyes a complimentary "fringe."

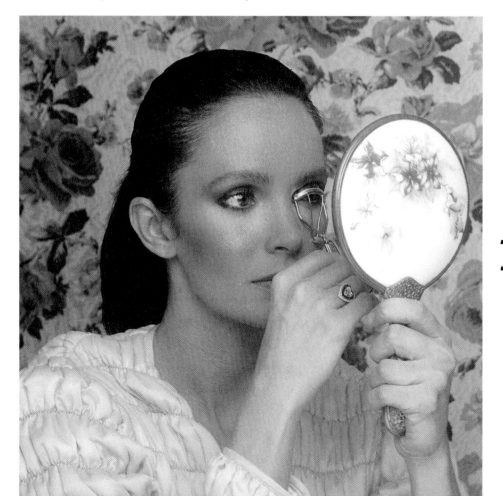

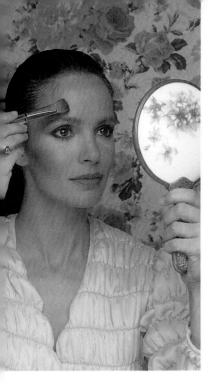

The gentlest contouring means blending a brown face powder across a broad forehead . . .

. . . and along the bottom edges of cheekbones.

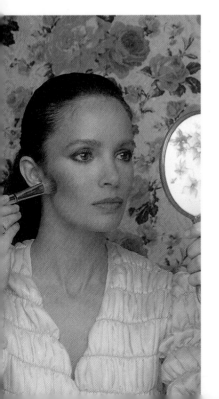

And I know they say that drawing a line around the eye makes it appear smaller, but I'm convinced the opposite is true. I think that lining really accentuates the eyes, which for so many women are their best feature—certainly their most expressive.

It is definitely laziness that's brought me to eyelash dyeing. I have an expert dye them black (only the fairest redheads and blondes need choose brown lashes) with a natural vegetable dye, about once every six weeks or so. This way, I don't ever have to think about mascara for daytime wear. But for those of you who do wear it, I can't really recommend colored mascaras. What could be more unnatural than navy blue or magenta hair? It helps set the mascara if you powder between applications. And when the mascara is dry, use that marvelous little invention, a lash curler, just to perk them up a bit. Then, apply a bit more mascara to set the new sweep.

I'm in the process of letting my eyebrows grow out into an almost completely natural state. That way, I won't have to worry about plucking them, except to keep them tidy. But I don't believe in pencil-thin brows or tortured arcs. A woman's natural brow is often the most flattering accent to her eyes.

Naturally, if you have seriously overwhelming brows, plucking or even waxing may be the answer. Too-dark brows can easily, and safely, be lightened, too—something women who color their hair should consider. The few stray hairs across the bridge of the nose or along the browbone can be controlled with occasional plucking, or tweezing.

I wear brow pencil only on a film set, but I can see how color applied in gentle, hairlike strokes can fill in any thin spots and can help add definition to too-pale or wispy brows.

FACE SHAPING

During the day, if I wear cheek color at all, it's a peachy powder-blush shade. I was born with a lot of color in my cheeks and find that for just being around the house or for everyday activities, I can skip it altogether. When I do have to look more pulled together, or for work under bright lights, day or night, I've learned to do a little subtle contouring first, to give a few angles to my basically oval face. (Now that my face appears thinner since Gaston's birth, I have to be very careful not to overdo the contouring.)

Because I have a rather broad forehead, I brush a warm brown powder all along the hairline, down to the temples and around the browbone, on both sides, of course. Next, it goes on just along the bottom edge of my cheekbones, creating the suggestion of a hollow, and under my chin, blended down the neck. Even at my age, it's unbelievably important to shade the neck, especially for film or television work!

If your face is more square in shape, you might want to skip the contouring along the hairline and concentrate on the temples and that hollow under the cheekbones. For you, neck contouring could be less important than carefully shading the back of the jawbone on either side, to soften the somewhat squarish shape.

Women with triangular or heart-shaped faces would be concerned about narrowing, that is, shading slightly darker, the widest part of the face, at the temples and in front of the ears.

The illusion of narrowing a too-large or too-wide nose can be created by contouring, too, but it must be done skillfully. Apply the brown powder (or you can use a cream blush, if you find that easier to handle) to either side of the nose, and blend completely. If the shading is left too dark, it'll look as if you've been staying up too late or been in a fight, rather than playing down a slight imperfection.

Always keep in mind the principle that darkened areas appear to recede while lightened ones leap forward to the observer's eye. Thus, the key to successful contouring is blending, either with a brush, or if you're using a cream formulation, with a sponge. There must be no lines of demarcation or the whole face-defining, accenting effect is spoiled.

Next to go on is the blush, just at the center of each cheek. I smile at myself in the mirror and brush the color onto the protruding apples of my cheeks and then thoroughly blend it into the brown contouring powder with a fresh makeup brush.

Finally, I dust with translucent face powder. I prefer a sheer powder that allows my skin's natural glow to come through. I'm not after a completely matte finish.

LUSCIOUS LIPS

·

By day, I often just wear a clear-pink gloss over a soothing, softening lip cream. That's partly because I have a lot of natural color in my lips already, and partly because I don't like a heavily made-up mouth. I think a glossy, but not sticky, look is prettier, even sexier.

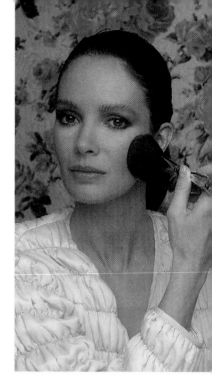

The finishing face touch: a dusting with translucent powder

To define the mouth, start with concealer blended all around the lips.

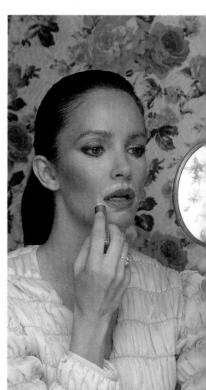

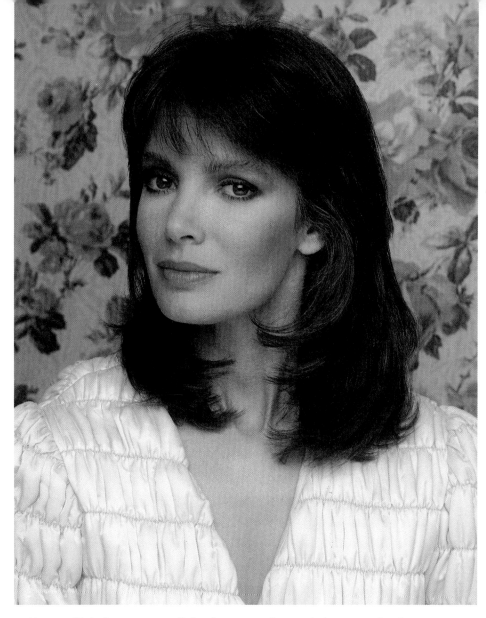

For a slightly more polished, more dressed daytime look, I use my concealer stick all around the edge of my lips. It gives heightened definition to the mouth, before the addition of lip color.

SPECIAL EFFECTS

At night, if Tony and I are going out, or having a dinner party at home, I love to do something a little more dramatic with my makeup. For instance, I might line my eyes on the *inside* of the lower rim—in cobalt blue—for a real standout effect. And I also put on black, lash-thickening, wand mascara—yes, over my already-dyed lashes!

For added after-dark glamour, I sometimes dot a little surprise of

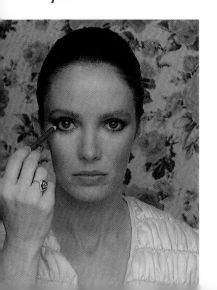

color on my eyelids—a lavender, blue, or pretty pink—just at the center, over the pupil. I also might shade the crease of the eyelid with brown shadow, blended subtly all the way up into the brow. And when I apply my pencil liner, I tend to extend it out about a half inch beyond the edge of each eye, in a gentle, upward stroke, for another lift.

The brown and peach contour/blush approach is the same, but for evening, I like to add a third color: a real pink. It goes on just at the apples of my cheeks, along the tops of my cheekbones, over the peach, and I touch it to the outside edge of the browbones, toward my temples, too. Using a bright pink this way, above the eyes, is amazingly effective as a highlighter. It can make your eyes positively compelling!

Although I'm not a big fan of high iridescence when it comes to makeup, at night I do sometimes use eye shadows with a hint of shine. And I invariably select a shimmery lipstick, a pink or even a real red, with a touch of gold or silver in it.

Lip liner comes into play, for me, when I'm making up for the evening. It's particularly helpful in shaping any irregularities in my lip line that may show up when I'm wearing real color on my lips. Sometimes I use pencil lip liner in the same shade as the lipstick I've chosen to wear. Other times, I'll line *and* color my lips with one pencil. Why not?

I think nighttime is the right time to experiment with less conservative makeup colors and applications and to have some fun playing with all the latest fashion shades. I don't offer any color-chart rules, because every woman's eye coloring, shape of face and eyes are so different. What's right for me might be totally wrong for you. But if it's special-occasion makeup, I say, "Go for it." Try out that eye shadow you bought and have been keeping in a drawer. You simply have to be prepared to remove it and start again if it doesn't flatter your individual face and your tastes.

Day or night, the single most significant thing is that makeup never "read." That's a professional term meaning to stand out, seem too apparent. Makeup is meant to refine what's already there. That's why I'm always a little disappointed to see girls of thirteen and fourteen wearing full makeup. What's "already there" is so fresh and simple and lovely just as it is.

The highest compliment, to me, is when someone says, "Why, you don't wear any makeup at all!" That means the effort, the careful application and blending, has been worth it. When this happens, I smile, and enjoy a secret satisfaction. And I never contradict!

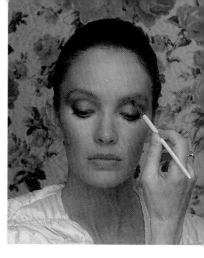

To heighten depth of eyes, shadow the crease with brown powder.

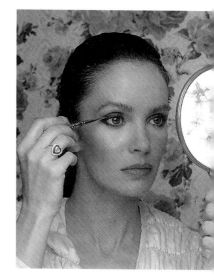

For after-dark wear, liner can be exaggerated—can be extended up and out from the corners of the eyes.

Line lips for definition and to correct any little imperfections.

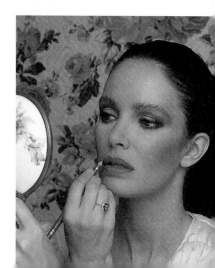

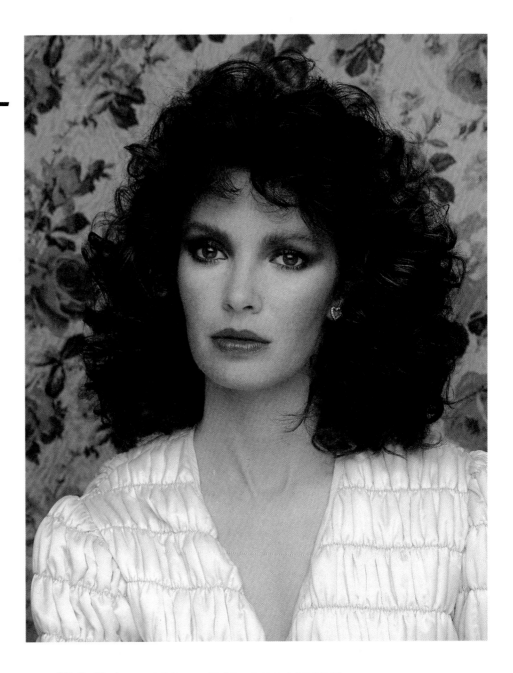

*A glamorous, yet
believable nighttime look*

V.S.O./VERY SPECIAL OCCASIONS

There are times in any woman's life—her wedding, or a very formal party—when she has to look her best, and does, usually with some professional help. In my life, when it comes to an Emmy Awards ceremony or dinner at the White House—an unforgettable night in the fall of 1983—it's "Call in the experts!"

I was, of course, thrilled at the President and Mrs. Reagan's invitation to attend a state dinner honoring Karl Carstens, the president of West Germany. I was, frankly, also quite panicked. I was between roles on the East and West coasts and had so little time to get ready. I needed help. But fortunately the designer Fabrice agreed to make me a fabulous beaded gown on short notice. And one of my favorite hairstylists, Emma di Vittorio, agreed to meet me in Washington, D.C., on the appointed evening. The makeup I handled myself.

Everything worked out as planned, and once made up, dressed and coiffed, I arrived at the White House feeling quite confident that I looked all right. In any case, Tony was at my side to give me even more confidence, but neither one of us knew what to expect.

As we entered the room where all the guests were gathering, I had a sense of coming into a different world—so stately and glamorous and powerful—but at the same time, I was struck by the warmth of it all. Tony and I felt as if we had been invited into the Reagans' living room, even though there were aides and waiters around everywhere to see that you had whatever you wanted.

Then we went into the main reception room, where we were introduced to the President, the First Lady and their guests from West Germany. The President was charming. And Mrs. Reagan made me feel completely relaxed during just a moment's greeting in the reception line.

You can imagine my delight in discovering, as we went on into the beautifully decorated dining room, that I was seated at a table for eight that included the First Lady as well as the German President and Helen Hayes. After dinner, we were escorted into another room for coffee, still another for entertainment and yet another for dancing. It really was a Cinderella evening. Never stuffy or overly formal, just enjoyably grand.

Most women, of course, can't summon dress designers and hairstylists for the very special occasions in their lives. But that's not the point. We should all do our very best, and then forget about it. Worrying about how you look is a real waste of time. You might miss something! That's why, once I arrive at a party, I forget about my looks. I can't stand women who constantly check themselves in a reflective surface or fuss with their hair. Nor do I think it's polite to whip out a compact and redo one's makeup or hair in public.

For a formal occasion, or even a restaurant dinner, I think all touch-up work should be reserved for the ladies' room. And I do mean touch-up; I'm just not interested in a major overhaul in the middle of a party. My evening bag contains only a lip gloss, for moisture more

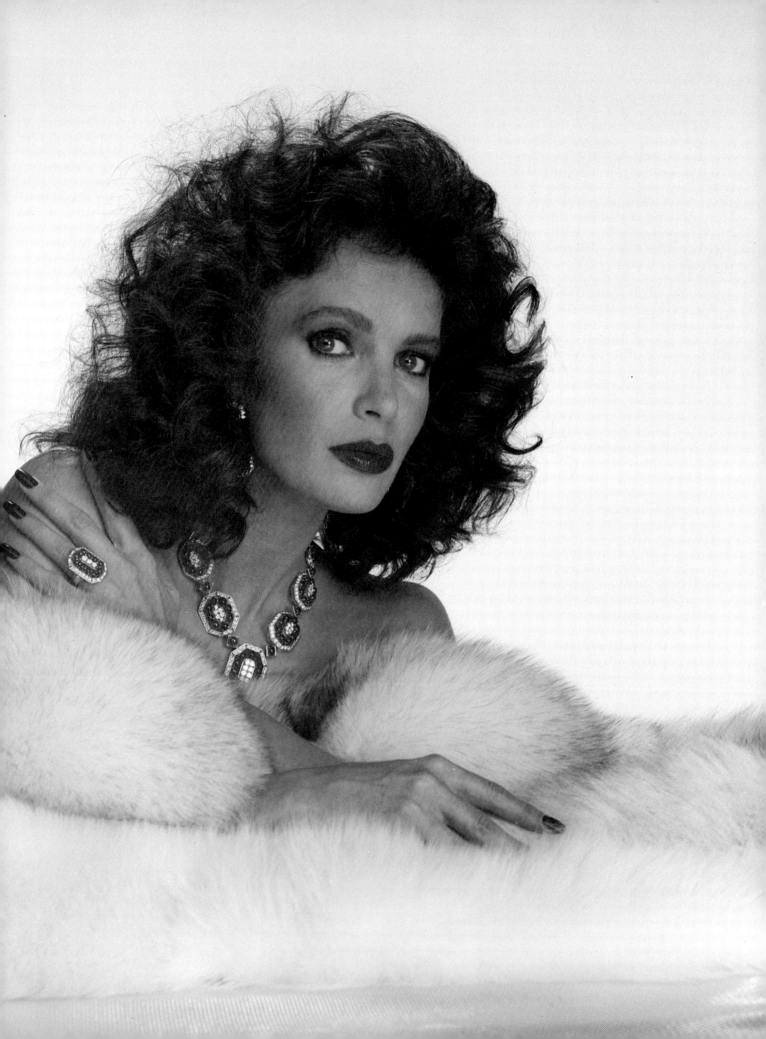

than for color or shine; an antique gold compact with a heart locket in its lid that my mother gave me, for unscented loose powder; a mini Mason Pearson hairbrush; a lace handkerchief tied around a little potpourri; and my key ring. That last item is always included because it has a picture of Gaston, at birth, on it. It's the kind of silly thing mothers cherish; I'm sure I'll still be carrying it when he's twenty!

MORE MAKEUP TIPS

- Makeup is meant to enhance; so decide—and only *you* can—which is your best feature, and play it up. You'll profit much more with this approach than in spending a great deal of time trying to mask a less attractive feature.

- If you've ever had the experience of making up, say, under the fluorescent light of a ladies' room, then being horrified by the effects once you get back to your office or out onto the street, you'll understand this piece of advice. Apply makeup in the same kind of light in which it will be seen. If you have no window in your bathroom, check your daytime look by outdoor light sometime *before* you go out. If you're going to a softly lit restaurant, dim the lights at your makeup table or in the bathroom and add more color. (You'll find your face can carry a lot more makeup in these cases.) But if a brightly lit ballroom is your destination, tone down the colors a bit.

- Ideally, leave yourself about twenty minutes to get dressed and do your hair, after you've finished putting on your makeup. Then go back and check it to see what you really have. Depending on the oiliness of your skin on any given day, the makeup may tend to sink in and disappear. You might want to freshen it up a bit before going out.

- Don't be shy about taking advantage of the tips you can pick up from department-store makeup artists and demonstrators. Almost every major city has a salon where you can go for a one-on-one makeup lesson. Many times you'll come away from a session like that with a lot of helpful information you can put to use, all by yourself, at home.

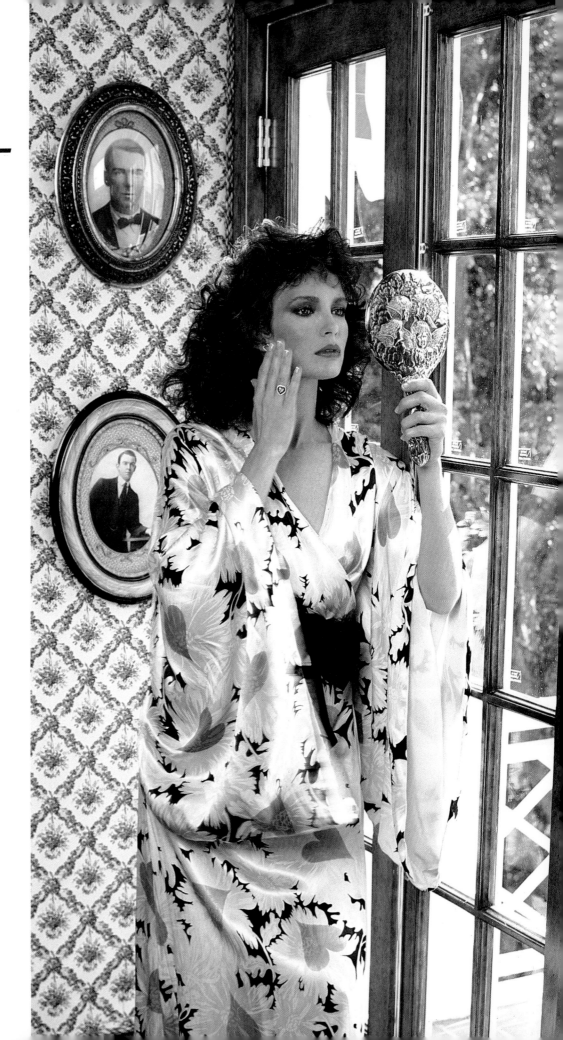

It's important to check your makeup in the same light in which you'll be seen. And remember, evening makeup is on view in sunlight during long summer days.

I wouldn't, on the other hand, let a professional give you a completely untried makeup look for a big evening. Just as with a brand-new hairstyle or gown, you're likely to feel a little unsure of it at first. Save this kind of enjoyable experimenting for a time when you can go straight home and assess and then adjust the look if necessary. But by all means, revisit a pro whose work you've appreciated for a V.S.O.

• When you travel as much as I do, it's a good idea to double up on favorite-makeup purchases—one for your bathroom at home and one for your travel case. In fact, it's not a bad idea for any working woman to have seconds handy for a purse or desk drawer. I just know how disappointed I am not to have *that* special lipstick with me when I want it or to discover that a shade I particularly like has been discontinued.

• My bias is obvious, but I happen to think my mother is one of the loveliest women I know. I've learned so much from her over the years—not the least of it, her light-touch attitude toward makeup. And lately, I've realized she's a perfect example of the mature woman's correct approach. Conventional wisdom may say that over-forty women should use paler makeup tones, but the fact is that deeper, more distinct colors—again, properly applied—give a face that's perhaps slightly less firm more dynamism and definition.

• From my work in television and films, I've become dependent on a professional, theatrical makeup product called Mellow Yellow. It's a great spot color corrector that blocks out red tones, and foundation is easily applied over it. If you're interested, you'll have to try beauty-supply houses. All I know is that no top-flight makeup artist would be caught dead without it.

• Any model or actress, or anyone who wears makeup for professional reasons, will agree with me that makeup removal, every night, no matter how tired you are, is critical. As pretty as all those colored powders and creams are, they can clog your pores and wreak havoc with your skin if left on overnight.
    Soap and water are all right; a light-textured makeup-removal cream or liquid, even gentler. And be certain to use a specially designed eye-makeup remover. Otherwise, the rubbing and scrubbing you do to this most tender of all areas will show over time.

I love the effects a good makeup job can achieve with any face. But while you're at it, in front of the mirror with all those marvelous powders and colored pencils waiting to make you beautiful, remember one thing: makeup is meant to enhance you, not transform you. A light touch and colors always blended well are the keys.

The Foundation

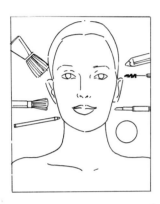

1. The canvas—your skin—should be clean and moisturized. Add a sunblock if your moisturizer or makeup foundation doesn't contain one and you're going to be outside in daylight.

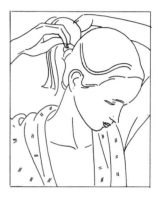

2. Wait for all the skin-care emollients to soak in. Why not pin back your hair or secure it in a headband while you're waiting?

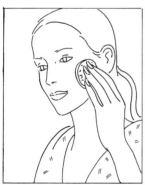

3. Correct a reddish or yellowish cast in your skin tone with a prefoundation color corrector; use green or mauve, respectively. Use a sponge for application.

4. Apply your foundation—chosen to match your natural skin tone within one shade—by dotting on—with fingertips—dime-sized blobs at the forehead, chin and on each cheek. (For ultrasheer coverage, dilute foundation with water.) Using a fresh sponge, blend carefully, gently, all over face and down onto the neck, so there's no line of demarcation.

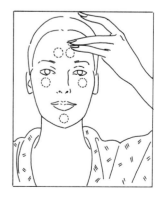

The Eyes

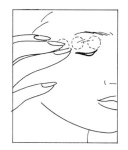

1. Prepare eyelids with a primer—either powder or an eye-shadow base, which you dot on your lids and blend with a fingertip.

2. Apply a specially formulated eye cream; allow to soak in.

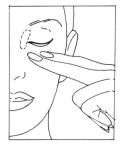

3. Dab on concealer stick, then blend thoroughly, around but not under the eyes, and in the usually dark hollows on either side of the nose. Choose a tone no more than one shade lighter than your foundation.

4. Line your eyes, just along the upper and lower lashes, with powder shadow, a pencil, or one of the new powder pencils. No need to choose a color that matches your eye shade. But do take the time to blend the line you've made into a subtle, eye-enhancing shadow line.

5. If you've not learned about the joys of eyelash dyeing, apply mascara, powdering between applications. Black's good for all but the fairest lashes; a dark brown is right in that case.

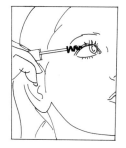

6. When mascara is dry, use a lash curler to fluff them up a bit. You might want to apply a second coat of mascara to set their new sweep.

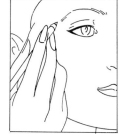

7. Fill in any thin spots in your brows with sketchy, hairlike strokes of a brow pencil in a matching shade. Otherwise, keep them plucked to neatness, in a basically natural line.

The Face

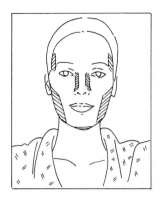

1. If you feel that contouring is necessary, use a neutral, brown-toned powder wherever you want to create the look of a hollow or indent. For instance, at the temples contouring can narrow and balance a top-heavy, heart-shaped face. The illusion of high cheekbones can be achieved with brown shadows added just along the bottom edge of the cheekbones. A vague jawline or chin can be made more distinct with a bit of contouring along the jaw and on the underneath plane of the chin. NOTE: None of this works if the contouring isn't blended down to the subtlest of shadows. Doing it well takes some practice.

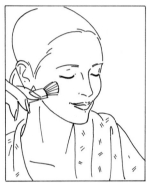

2. Apply blusher in a natural-looking shade of peach, pink, or rose to the apples of your cheeks. To find them, smile at yourself in the mirror and blush those little mounds that protrude.

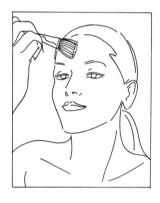

3. Finish with a light, allover dusting of transparent face powder to set your makeup and absorb any oiliness in hours to come.

The Lips

1. I always wear a soothing, softening lip balm, because there's nothing less appealing, not to mention uncomfortable, than chapped, dry-looking lips.

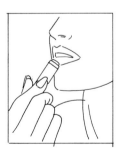

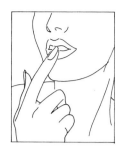

2. For informal daytime makeup, I'd suggest just a light glossing of the mouth with a transparent lip gloss, again in a natural pink, peach, or rose shade.

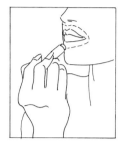

3. For more polish, try outlining your lips with your concealer stick before applying any lip color or gloss. This gives the mouth greater definition, more impact. Of course, the concealer is—need I say it?—completely blended.

Nighttime Glamour

There are many little tricks and tips you can use to glamorize your makeup at night, when a more made-up look is totally appropriate. Here are some of my favorites:

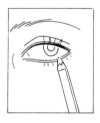

1. Line the *inside,* lower rims of your eyes with color—even cobalt blue!—for real impact. A pencil's the tool to choose for this technique. Alternatively, you could simply extend your daytime, smudged eyeliner color beyond the outside corners of the eyes and a bit upward for an after-dark lift.

2. Add to the defined structure of the eye by coloring the eyelid crease with a brown or gray shadow; finish by smudging the color ever so subtly up into the eyebrow.

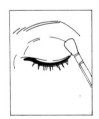

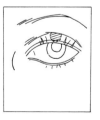

3. Dot a surprise of color—a lilac, pink, or even yellow—on the center of each eyelid. It mirrors the pupil and holds a viewer's attention.

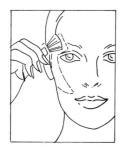

4. Use your regular blush—or a second, slightly brighter, "punchier" shade—to extend the wash of color from the apples of the cheeks, out along the cheekbones to the temples. Swing the color back around onto the browbone and blend completely.

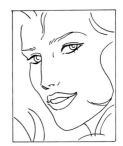

5. Night's the time to try out shimmery eye shadows and lipsticks, but be careful of anything with a too-white shine. Look for products with hints of gold or silver light instead.

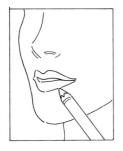

6. In addition to setting them up with the concealer stick, outline the mouth in a lip pencil that matches, or very nearly matches, your lip color.

CONVERSATION WITH AN EXPERT: DAVID FRANK RAY ON MAKEUP

David Frank Ray is a free-lance makeup artist who's worked with numerous actresses, celebrities and models in a career that spans print advertising, movies and commercials for television and many fashion-magazine layouts—both here and in Europe. I first met David when he was called to do my makeup for the supersuccessful "Charlie's Angels" poster of Kelly Garrett about four years ago. Here, I talk with David about some of the facts and fads in makeup.

JS: I know you like to use sponges for foundation application. What are your other favorite professional tools?

DFR: Yes, I do like the sponge for foundation makeup—when you're after everyday, light coverage—because you can use lots of water to dilute it, and it goes on easily and smoothly. For heavier coverage, though, I might dab on the foundation with a sponge, then use my fingertips to blend it. I find that something about the warmth of my skin really helps a heavier foundation adhere and blend better.

I have a range of superfluffy to more concentrated-bristle makeup brushes for applying powder blush and regular face powder. And for lips, I like to use a pencil to define the mouth and contain the fill-in lipstick. But I always use a Q-tip or lip brush to buff and soften the line of lip liner.

JS: What about tools for eye makeup? Do you prefer pencils, little brushes, or those sponge-tipped applicators?

DFR: The technique I find best for applying eye makeup involves lining *and* shading the eyelid with a pencil, then shading the eyelid again with the same or an interestingly contrasted powder shadow. I might use a navy pencil with purple shadow, for example, or gray with olive. For the shadow itself, I prefer those little brushes cut at an angle at the edge. That wedge-shaped edge lets you use the brush to stroke on color or to sort of dot it on.

JS: How do you care for these tools? Is it important to wash them often?

DFR: Oh, yes. It's like having a clean toothbrush that's in good shape. I've discovered a quick-dry cleanser for brushes and sponges that's made by Temporella. It's really like dry-cleaning them instead of washing. It's much quicker. But if you don't have that solution, you can always soak the applicators and brushes in Woolite. It's just that it takes them quite a while to dry thoroughly.

JS: You tend to double up on makeup formulations and colors, don't you? Like your use of pencil, then powder eye shadow.

DFR: Yes, I think doubling up like that can give you color depth that makes the finished makeup look real, as if it really comes from the face. For example, to give a real-life blush to the face, I first apply a cream blush, with my fingertips, then dust with a sheer powder; even baby powder will do. That way, any oil on the skin or from the cream blush is set. Then I brush on a powder blush in the same, or a very similar, color, right over everything. I finish with an allover dusting of transparent face powder.

I double up on the lips by starting with a liner pencil to strengthen and define the mouth. Then I fill in with a lipstick as close to the same

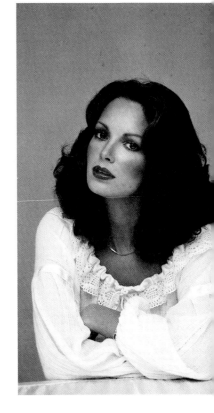

My Charlie's Angel look required a light but sure touch in applying makeup.

shade as possible. The matching of lip pencil to lipstick is the key to avoid a strange, two-toned look.

JS: In general, where do you apply blusher?

DFR: The cream blush I'll blend into the cheeks, up toward the temples. But I don't like the final look to be one of two balanced blotches of color on either side of the nose. So I brush the second-phase powder blush up onto the browbone, over the eye makeup, as well as a touch on the chin, across the forehead. Using that same hint of color all over seems to pull the whole face together.

JS: How should a woman choose makeup shades? By considering her hair color? Her skin tone? The latest fashion?

DFR: I happen to believe that almost any woman can wear some variation on any color. Sure, there are some tonalities of pink that suit a blond's usually white/fair skin tone better than a redhead's. But beyond skin tone, what the women will be wearing is the determining factor.

JS: I think most women feel—rightly—that their eyes are their best feature. What are your tricks for making eyes look big and beautiful?

DFR: I think mascara is unbelievably important in creating alluring eyes. Black mascara, and the use of an eyelash curler, are great boons to any face.

Then you have to analyze your particular situation. If, for instance, a woman has eyelids that protrude, she'll want to choose a darker rather than a lighter shadow for that area, to make it recede. If the eye has no lid showing when it's open, it's dead wrong to use a highlighter on that browbone area. What you want is a soft brown or something deeper to focus the viewer's attention away, to the eye itself.

As far as lining the eye goes, if you have small or narrow eyes, lining them all the way around will only make them appear smaller. In fact, for most women, it's best to line the eye only from the center of the lid out to the corner—and then along the bottom lashes, from the corner back nearly to the center of the eye. There is, however, a trendy new look that does call for just lining the top lid, and it can be flattering. To make the eye appear bigger and wide-set you also want to widen the lining at the outside corners, ending up with a sort of smudged, mini-pyramid shape of color.

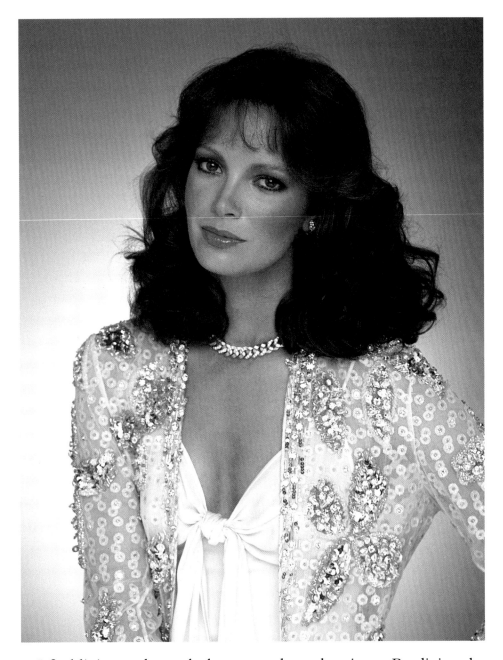

I find lining underneath the eye tends to close it up. But lining the lower rim of the eye—on the *inside*—with white eye pencil, instead of the now old-fashioned cobalt blue or kohl colors, does tend to open and enlarge the eyes.

JS: Do you use a lot of frosted or iridescent makeups?

DFR: I'm adamant that iridescence is not a daytime look. But at night, when you're going to be seen under softer, lower lighting, I might dot a little silver, pink, or gold, like a spotlight, over the pupil, under the browbone or on the inside corners of the lids to add an appealing glow to the face.

JS: Does it please you to think that women study and try to emulate the makeup looks you've done for celebrities and models in ads and movies?

DFR: Of course I'm pleased when people admire my work. But what I do professionally is often just fantasy, meant to inspire people, to get them to experiment with their own faces, but never meant to be taken literally. It's really a practical thing: those incredibly hot and intense lights used in photography and filming require, usually, more makeup. Plus, the camera magnifies everything about a face. The whole thing bears no resemblance to the way a woman should look, walking down the street, in what I call "real life." Besides, each face is unique, and what I might do for you may not be correct for someone else.

I don't like to see a lot of makeup on a woman during the day. Cosmetics are, after all, only meant to enhance, not mask.

JS: At what age should girls start wearing makeup, in your opinion?

DFR: That's very tough to answer generally. I do believe that children are never too young to learn about good skin care, healthy cleansing and maintenance techniques. Then, when it comes to the "decoration," it really depends on the individual girl's interest level. You can start very young girls who want to wear makeup with little things, like lip balm as a clear lip gloss and a little baby powder to tone down any oiliness or shine. But you can also give them a lip brush and a blusher/powder brush to put them on with. That way, they become familiar with proper application. Later, when they're introduced to real cosmetics, they'll have a better understanding of their use.

JS: What should mature women change about their makeup? Should they wear more or less, darker or lighter colors?

DFR: Everything starts to blur a bit as women get older: the face loses color; the features become less distinct. I think the whole makeup should be a little more defined, cleaner, clearer.

Foundation should still match the skin tone as closely as possible and be applied in a very sheer layer. Then, brush on face powder to minimize wrinkles. Eyes need more definition than ever, too, so mascara, use of the curling wand and lining are especially important. I don't think you want a lot of color on the eyes. Certainly not anything muddy or pastel. Soft neutrals like charcoal and rust are best. And avoid iridescent shadows; they're drying and tend to heighten any wrinkling or crepiness of the skin.

The lip pencil's important, again for increased definition. And now there are several good products out, designed to help keep lipstick color from fading into the little wrinkles that often form around the lips. And again, you'd want a soft but clear color. Not the dusty, dramatic browns, the reddest reds, or frosted pales that a younger woman can get away with. Keep your blush in the same tone as lips, but think about using a cream-blush formulation to avoid a dried-out look.

JS: What are the makeup mistakes women make most often?

DFR: The first offender is always a lack of proper, complete blending. We talked about tools, but I neglected to mention one special brush—the bristles are fairly tightly packed, and the brush part is about one-and-a-half to two inches long—that I keep separate for blending the makeup at the end. I go over the whole face to blend and smudge out any "edges."

Otherwise, women tend to wear too much or too little makeup. Either they're afraid of it and have given up altogether, or they've gone overboard. That's why I don't recommend that women try contouring on their own, unless they've had some professional help in learning how to do it properly. So many times I spot women who are, for instance, trying to camouflage a prominent nose. But they've done the contouring awkwardly, or not blended it enough, and the result calls attention to that feature. Exactly the opposite of the goal.

If you have a feature you don't like, I think it's safer and wiser to leave it matte and sort of ignore it, in favor of another feature you want to enhance.

The only exception to that rule is a kind of contouring for the neck. Any puffiness that threatens to grow into a double chin, or any lack of definition at the jawline can be remedied with a bit of blush. Just a dash of powder blush in a soft, brown tone under the chin, with the transparent face powder blended over it, works like subtle contouring.

CONVERSATION WITH AN EXPERT: DR. JACK SMITH ON YOUR SMILE

One thing any successful model or actress simply cannot live without is a beautiful smile. Dr. Jack Smith, a practicing dentist for some fifty-five years, is largely responsible for my smile. As well as being my father, he's my dentist. And here he shares with me his tenets for achieving and maintaining that perfect smile.

JS: I think everybody's stereotype of a Hollywood smile is a mouthful of capped teeth. Is that the only way to get a camera-perfect smile?

DR. S: The technique for applying caps used to involve a lot of pressure on the teeth underneath, so that they were usually reserved for front teeth only. Now there do exist ways to get a whole mouth capped. But I have to say, they're not always that well done. I can tell, even on television, when someone has caps. The real advances now are in a technique called acid etching.

JS: How does that work?

DR. S: Instead of drilling or filling the existing imperfect teeth, they are treated with a weak acid that creates microscopic porosities. Then toothlike material is applied to fill in gaps or chips.

JS: Is that what you did for me?

DR. S: That's right. You had a good occlusion, or bite, but a slight defect: a gap, or diastema, between your two front teeth. It could have been corrected with an orthodontic appliance, but when the doctor told you how long you'd have to wear it, you weren't very pleased. So we went with the dental etch, which has remained in fabulous shape. The color's quite stable. It's given very good results.

JS: I think it was model/actress Lauren Hutton who made those clip-in gap-fillers widely known. What are their drawbacks?

DR. S: Those plastic gap-fillers you can clip in and out can come loose just when you're talking or eating. People often lose them or swallow them. When I have my dental lab make one up for a patient, I order three or four at a time, knowing some are bound to be lost.

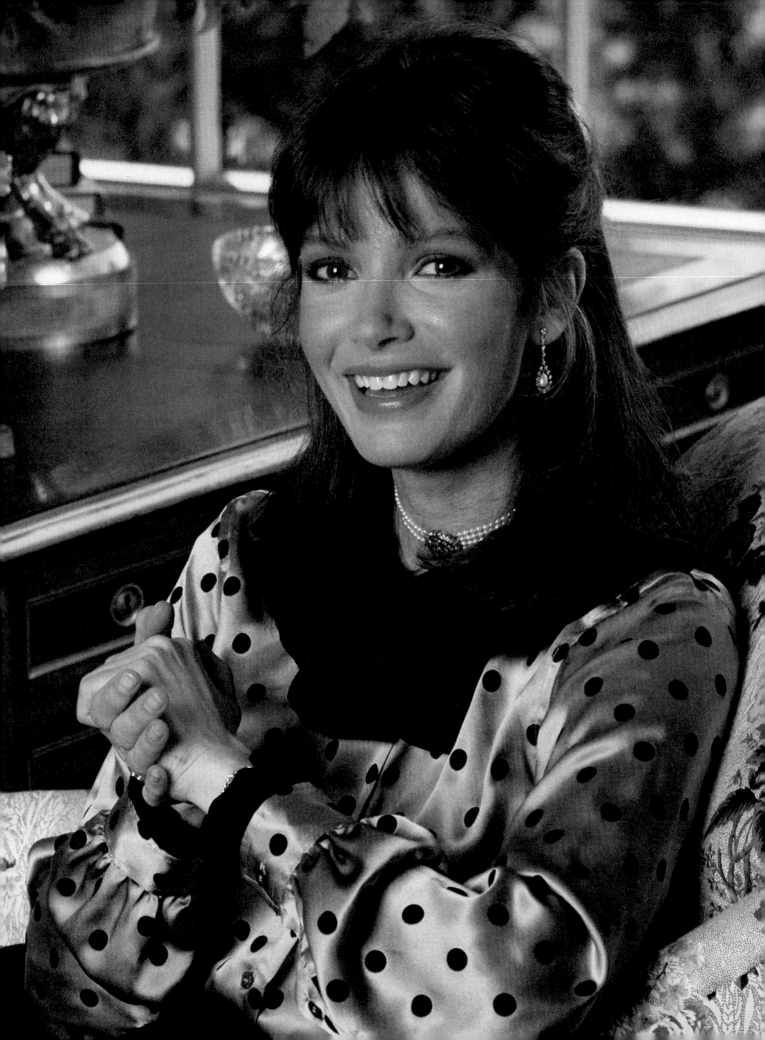

Needless to say, you don't have that problem with the acid etch. Plus, your own teeth aren't filed, so you don't become what I call a dental cripple.

JS: Generally, are you in favor of adult orthodontics?

DR. S: I believe it's never too late. But now my interest in straightening teeth is so they become easier to clean, therefore easier to preserve. I'm not so much interested in the cosmetic effects. But I have patients in their fifties and sixties with orthodontic appliances.

JS: What are your guidelines for maintaining good teeth?

DR. S: It's hardly revolutionary advice, but I'd say brushing as many as three times a day, using dental floss regularly and seeing your dentist.

JS: Is there a right way to brush?

DR. S: Well, there are many theories. But I still brush the way my professor at Baylor University taught me. And I still have my teeth even though I'm getting up there in age!

His method is to hold the brush at a forty-five-degree angle to the teeth, starting with the bristles mostly on the gums. Then you brush downward onto the chewing surface, covering about two or three teeth at a time. Repeat five times per section.

When you get to the tight spots, the anterior teeth on top, in front, you can only cover about one to one-and-a-half teeth at a time, using about three of the brush's top rows of bristles.

JS: How do you feel about the use of water-jet tooth-cleaning machines?

DR. S: I think they're great. In fact, when they first came out, I ordered about four hundred of them for my patients. They're particularly good for gum deterioration, but they are *never* a substitution for thorough brushing. Just a good ancillary treatment.

JS: What about brushing with baking soda? Is that a good idea?

DR. S: It's a perfectly good idea. You couldn't overdo it. You just mix a little baking soda with a few drops of peroxide to make a paste.

This is especially effective for people with gum problems, gums that bleed. It toughens up the gums.

JS: Do you recommend tooth-polishing and whitening products to be used at home?

DR. S: I don't have too much experience with them, but it seems to me that any product that could remove tobacco stains, say, at home, might be too harsh, too abrasive. As far as whitening agents are concerned, it's been my experience that nature usually provides teeth of a proper color to go with the person's complexion. Even a slight, naturally yellowish tint often suits the person's skin tone.

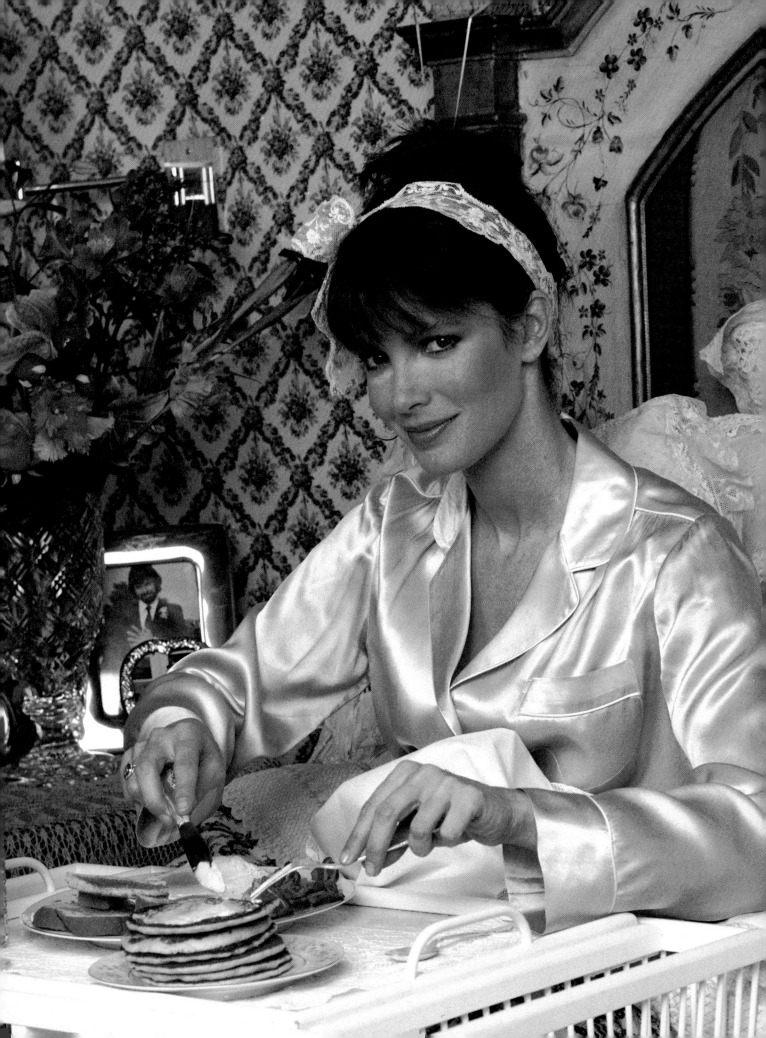

CHAPTER 7

Eating Well Is the Best Revenge

*I*f you've been hoping to read that I was a fat, dumpy child who dieted herself into sylphlike slimness, I'm sorry to have to disappoint you. Since early childhood, I've been thin, and in high school, I had to have protein drinks to keep me from becoming really too skinny. But as I've grown older, and had a child, I've learned to pay a lot more attention to my weight and nutrition, and their roles in my looks and my energy level.

YOU ARE WHAT YOUR MOTHER FEEDS YOU

I don't think there's any question that eating habits are developed very early in life. I grew up in Houston, with a mother who is a very good cook, and I ate three quite substantial, four-food-group meals a day.

Even as a very little girl, I had a huge breakfast, with my mother there to cook it for me every morning before school. It remains my favorite meal, and I support wholeheartedly the doctors who recommend a solid breakfast as essential to a weight-maintenance or even a weight-loss plan. It gives you the energy you need for the day; it sort of sets you up for anything that's ahead.

I carried my lunch to school, and it always included a huge bag of crisp, fresh carrot and celery sticks, an apple or other piece of fruit, as well as a sandwich and a soft drink. I feel so lucky now that I really *like* those vegetables others consider diet food; it's the crunchy dimension that has such an appeal.

Our dinners consisted of a lot of beef—much more than I eat these days; somehow, it tasted better to me then—or chicken, as well as fresh vegetables and salads. Great Southern dishes like spoon bread, fried okra, red pinto beans and grits were often part of the mix, too —and I did eat sweets. Just like any other kid, I had the occasional popsicle or ice cream cone and went to the store to buy suckers and candy bars. But I never became addicted, so sweets have never represented the great temptation for me that they are for so many women.

I must say that physically, I was always very active and agile. I ran in school, but eschewed other sports like hockey and tennis for my first love, ballet. Dancing was my favorite activity, and I studied it quite religiously from age three onward. (That song from *A Chorus Line,* "Everything Is Beautiful at the Ballet," could have been my theme!) But I've always enjoyed a metabolism that could deal with all the food I ate. As I mentioned, in high school they were worried I'd become too thin, even for a ballet dancer!

SENSIBLE EATING VERSUS STARVATION

Despite my good fortune in having little trouble maintaining my ideal 115 pounds at five feet seven inches, as a wife and mother involved in a very looks-oriented business, I'm constantly aware of what I, and my family, eat.

I'm still a breakfast fanatic, and that means juice, eggs, toast, coffee, the works! What I have for lunch depends so much on what's going on around me. If I'm working on the set, I find I can't possibly skip the midday meal. I need it to keep my energy up. So I might have a sandwich or some chicken or something like that from the catering truck, or I might send out for Italian food, or pizza, or hamburgers. I know this may sound dangerously like junk food, but if you think about it, a good hamburger with lettuce and pickles and all that great stuff is really quite a nutritious meal. And pizza with cheese, mushrooms, green peppers—anything but anchovies!—is reasonable too. It's just a question of not overdoing any of it.

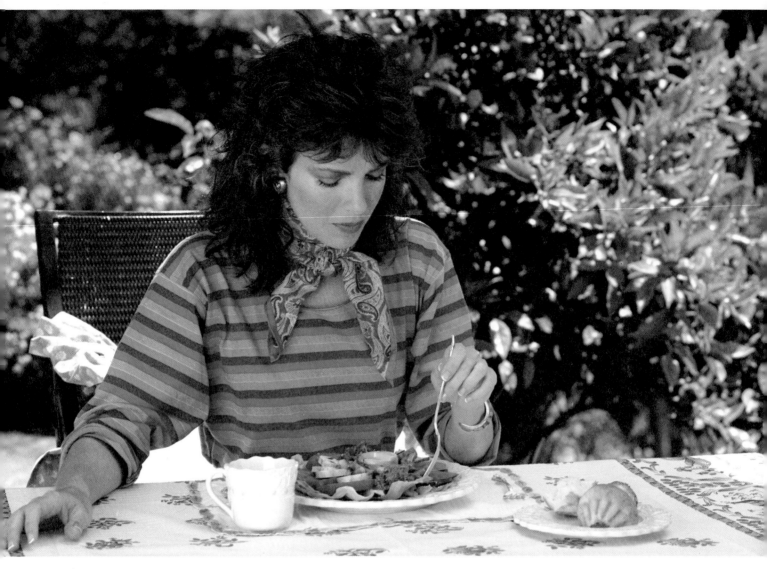

If I'm at home, I might skip lunch altogether, except for an apple or slices of papaya, which I love. Or, I'll fix a little healthful sandwich and eat with Gaston. Two of my favorite combinations are tuna (packed in water) mixed up with just a touch of lo-cal mayonnaise on plain matzo crackers—again, for texture—and a matzo with cheese melted over it, topped with sliced fresh tomato and a little mayonnaise.

Once in a while, I enjoy an icy Coca-Cola, but more often I choose a fructose-sweetened fruit drink. There's a brand called Hansen's available on the West Coast that comes in delicious flavors like lemon-lime, grapefruit and mandarin-lime; they even have a natural cola one

Good food, attractively presented, makes eating right easy.

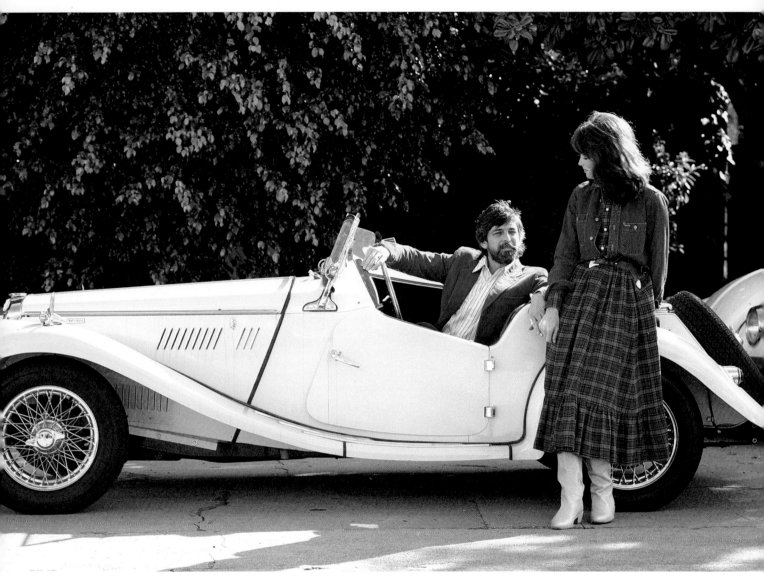

now. And since my pregnancy, I've made a concerted effort to keep up with the then-recommended eight glasses of water a day. I'd heard about this recommendation all my life but was never moved to try it until I was pregnant with Gaston. I'm now a believer. It cuts my appetite and helps rid my body of fluids so that I don't feel or look bloated.

I will admit, on the other hand, that some days it's hard to remember all eight, or to choke them down, but I've gotten into a pretty consistent routine. One glass of distilled or even tap water first thing in the morning; another midmorning; another before, then after lunch; two during the afternoon, one before dinner and a final glass before bed. Whew! But it works!

Tony is the cook, or rather, gourmet chef, around our household, so dinners are pretty interesting. I love ethnic cuisines, and he's adept at all of them—Italian, Mexican, Chinese, even soul food. But his real specialty is fine French food, and I'm more than happy to eat that, too!

I don't eat a lot of desserts, but, on the other hand, I don't deny myself a cookie or two, or a little ice cream if I feel like it. That kind of denial, on a regular basis, makes women agitated and angry, I think. I'm much more in favor of giving in to a whim every now and then, and perhaps making up for it by having a cleansing day afterward.

I call mine "purifying days" and stick adamantly to good things: fruits, vegetables, veal, or chicken. But I never starve myself.

When Tony and I go out to a restaurant—which, between our two busy schedules, is not often—I order whatever I like, especially since I never go out for lunch. It's just not a habit I developed. My favorite thing is to go to a great Italian restaurant, where I start with pasta, then a veal dish, usually a Caesar salad (without anchovies!) and maybe even a bite of some fabulous dessert. Other times, I'm attracted to the idea of a wonderful, hot cream soup—the kind my mother used to make, and now Tony, when he has the time. So you see, in general, my food style has remained plain, not picky.

NOTES ON NUTRITION AND DIET

- All this talk about food brings to mind the fact that food isn't everything. If you need to lose weight, almost all the professionals will tell you that dieting alone isn't the answer. A successful, long-term approach has to combine diet and some sort of exercise. That can be just walking—something I do a lot of—but some physical activity has to be part of the picture.

- I haven't yet consulted one, but I think the help of a professional nutritionist can be invaluable. Keeping a food diary, learning about particular food allergies and getting a lifetime eating plan sounds like fun to me.

- I've smoked a cigarette exactly once in my life, for a scene. It didn't

JACLYN SMITH'S WEIGHT-CONTROL PURIFYING DAY

Breakfast

- ½ grapefruit, 1 large orange, or ¾ cup strawberries; no sugar
- herbal tea

Lunch

- ¼ lb. white chicken meat; 1 sliced apple

  or

- ¼ lb. water-packed, white tuna meat, with a dab of lo-cal mayonnaise; 1 plain matzo
- iced caffeine-free tea

  or

- a fructose-sweetened fruit drink

Dinner

- paillard of veal, broiled, with lemon and pepper

  or

- 1 skinless chicken breast, broiled
- ½ cup of steamed broccoli, carrots, string beans, or zucchini; no butter
- water ★

★ These are the days I'm very conscious of drinking my eight glasses of water. (Herbal tea and decaffeinated coffee count, too!)

—and still doesn't—appeal to me, and I simply can add my warnings and concerns to those any smoker has heard again and again. I attribute my total lack of interest, by the way, to my passion for ballet. That one cigarette made me realize how smoking cuts down on one's wind, one's lung power, and that was enough for me.

- Though I've taken vitamins at various periods in my life—most consistently when I was pregnant—I've never established a viable, obviously effective pattern. But I'd like to. Here's another area where I think a nutritionist could help a great deal.

As it is, I take a Theragran tablet daily, when I remember to. Because I think vitamins are useful in combating the effects of our stressful modern lives, as well as for good physical health, I intend to develop a vitamin plan that works for me.

• Alcohol is another beauty spoiler that I've been blessed with a distaste for. I mean it. Even in college, I never went in for beer and wine parties in the dorm. My eyes were fixed on New York City, where I wanted to start acting or dancing, and alcohol just wasn't a part of that picture.

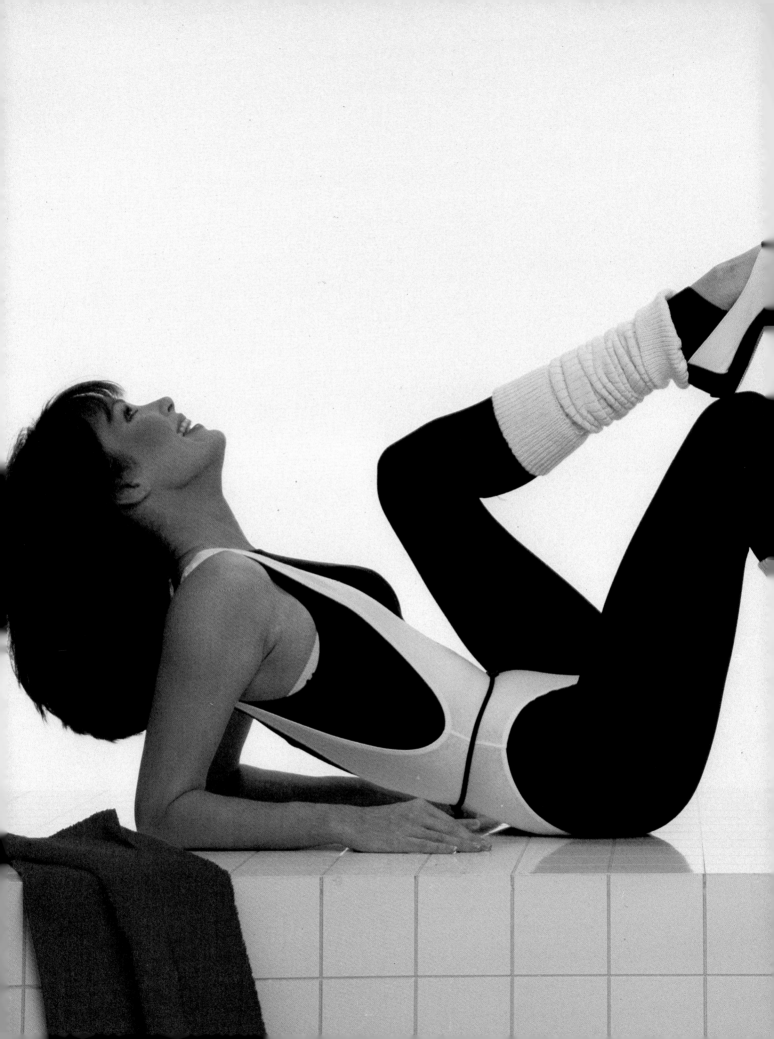

CHAPTER 8

Getting and Staying in Shape

I've always been vitally interested in keeping fit, and I've been active all my life. But it was through a radio program★ I narrated that I learned the facts about fitness. A lot of what you need to know is just good common sense.

First of all, let's get one thing straight: fitness and exercise aren't the same thing. You can exercise without getting fit, but you can't get fit without exercise. A little confused? It's just that the truest measure of how fit you are is the rate and efficiency of your cardio-vascular system. Other systems count, too, but your heart is your number one fitness priority.

Not all forms of exercise are equal in their benefits to your cardio-vascular system, either. Sit-ups, for instance, are great for toning your abdominal muscles, but they're not going to raise your heart rate. Lifting weights will increase your strength, but it won't give you greater endurance.

The real get-fit exercises are those that will raise your heart rate

★ An ABC radio series called "Alive and Fit."

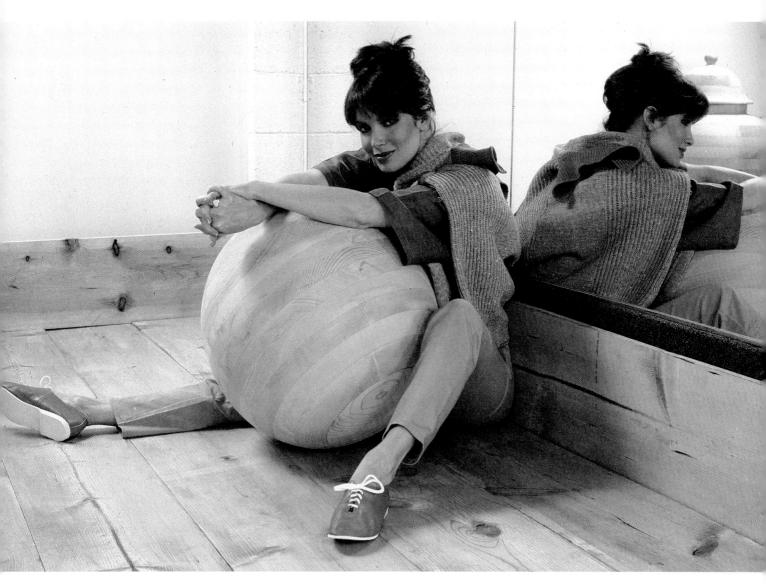

over a period of time—those exercises now known as aerobics. And they can be anything from brisk walking to dancing to swimming.

Fitness and thinness aren't synonymous, either. Your body needs calories from a balanced diet, *and* exercises for overall conditioning, for you to look and feel your best. But two women of the same height, given inescapable differences in bone and muscle structure as well as metabolic rate, can carry differing absolute weights and still be fit. The point here is to strive for fitness, not thinness. Fit *is* beautiful, by definition.

Fitness means increased energy, because your body is better able to take in oxygen and convert it to physical work than when you're in poor condition. It means that your heart's rate (your pulse) slows because you're in good condition, and at the same time, it's able to beat with greater force and pump more blood with each beat. Your lungs can take in and hold more air. Sounds rather appealing, doesn't it?

SO, WHERE TO BEGIN

Designing a good allover fitness program requires that you take into account all your body's needs, beginning with flexibility.

We've all heard that we're supposed to warm up before any kind of exercise or sport. And, with my dancer's training, I've acquired the habit of including warm-ups and cool-downs automatically. So should you—to avoid injury during exercise or any sports activity. But did you also realize that flexibility is an end in itself? Toning and endurance activities tend to build short muscles if those same muscles aren't stretched out before and afterward. That's what happens to some weight lifters when they become, literally, muscle-bound. So, begin your fitness routine with a few minutes of stretching and calisthenics.

Next comes aerobics. Skipping rope, running, swimming, or any variety of continuous effort maintained for at least twenty minutes qualifies as aerobics. Finally, do some weight training, for strength and balance among your muscles, to round out the ideal program. If you really want an overall fitness regimen, this is the best formula.

EXERCISE AND WEIGHT LOSS

Yes, some exercises are more effective than others when it comes to weight loss, because those exercises are better at increasing your body's loss of fat. Walking and jogging are particularly good choices, since they require you to put out a relatively low intensity of energy over a relatively long duration.

Low-intensity, long-duration activity uses calories and tones your muscles, but it doesn't deplete the stores of glycogen in your muscles and liver. That's important, because more vigorous, strenuous exercise tends to use up that stored glycogen, increasing, often, your appetite level. Since exercise, *plus* a lowered-calorie intake, is the ideal for slimming, such low-intensity activities can make it easier for you to stick to your diet.

Some people are quick to blame a "slow metabolism" for their inability to lose unwanted weight. And it is true that overweight people have slower metabolic rates, on average, than thin people. But here comes the Catch-22: it's *being* overweight that causes a slowdown in your body's metabolic rate. Not the other way around!

An active workout burns up calories and turns up your body's metabolism. In fact, your metabolic rate is raised for as much as four to six hours *after* you've finished your workout. With regular exercise, even if you don't alter your diet, you should burn more calories and lose weight. Now, do you see any way left to argue yourself out of exercise?

Another note: one exercise myth many of us have fallen for is the notion that working up a good sweat means we're losing weight. Wrapping yourself in plastic or nonbreathing, synthetic running suits can make you feel as if you're working harder. But the fact is, you're only working hotter. Sweating more doesn't mean you're burning off more of that unwanted fat. And overdoing it can be dangerous, causing fatigue, and in extreme cases, heat stroke.

CHOOSE YOUR PASSION

So, you've got the word about warming up. Now it's time to decide which exercise(s) and sport(s) will make up your personal-fitness regimen. This may come as a shock, but the single most significant factor in this decision ought to be that you choose activities you enjoy. Seriously. For the simple reason that, if you actually dread the weekly tennis game, you're eventually going to give it up.

I'm lucky that my lifelong love affair with dance—ballet and jazz and tap since age twelve—has always provided a fitness activity I truly adore. To this day, I can give myself a ballet class in a hotel room. And that training has made me experienced at being and staying aware of my body—its developing strengths and weaknesses. I've learned to tell what needs work and what doesn't. I wish each of you could find something as satisfying and healthful.

To that end, let me remind you that your fitness regimen doesn't have to be focused on just one thing. There are so many different forms of exercise and amusing sports to choose from. In addition to loving dance, I'm a pretty good water skier, have done a bit of snow skiing and like swimming. So no matter where I am in the world, there is some fitness-maintenance activity I can do.

One perfectly acceptable option is walking. Yes, simple, brisk walking is a safe and easy way to get exercise. For the more adventurous, there's also race walking, a speed sport that's much less hard on

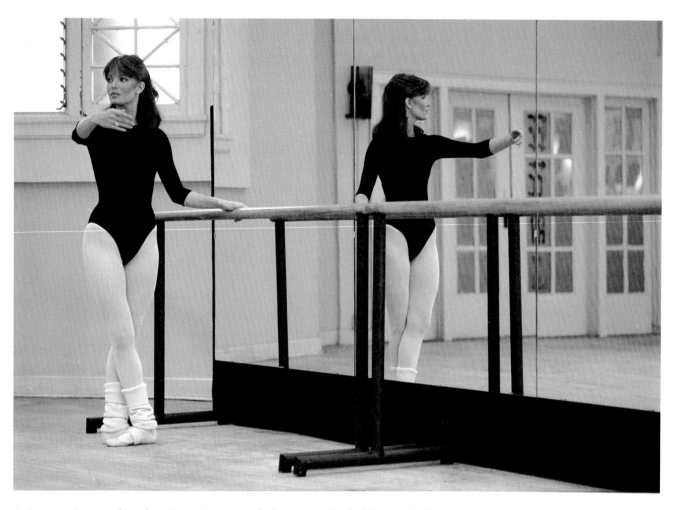

joints and muscles than jogging. And that cute little hip-swivel action involved in proper race walking helps cut down on bouncing, reducing the shock to your body when feet impact on a hard surface.

Racquet sports like tennis and racquetball are terrific for hand-eye coordination and—if you run a lot to meet the ball—your cardiovascular health. Racquetball has the advantage, in contrast with tennis—of being playable by oneself and is a sport wherein a beginner can burn up to 350 calories in an hour. Drawbacks with racquet sports are obvious: you tend to work only one side of your upper body muscles. But that's okay. Play your favorite racquet sport but add another exercise that'll offer a balance for the upper body—gymnastics, for example.

Yoga and ballet class are also fine choices, especially for the flexibility we've been talking about. Aerobic dance class and jogging are great choices for cardiovascular fitness.

In terms of the latter—running or jogging—it's key to keep in mind

A ballet workout is still my favorite way to keep stretched and fit.

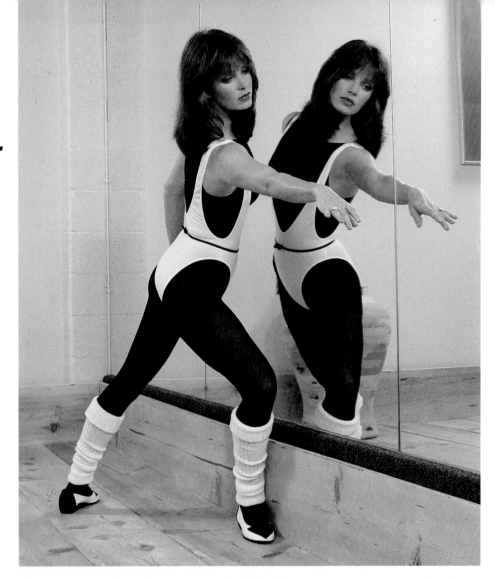

Ballet is great for flexibility, posture and grace.

that everyone has her own style. You'll see some runners take long strides, others short steps. Some run bolt upright, while others seem to lean forward. Whatever your style, there are some across-the-board caveats: run relaxed, with your body erect, not slumped down into your pelvis. Use your arms to give you balance and power as you run; don't let them hang at your sides like extra weights. And be sure to run or jog so that the heel of your foot strikes the pavement or track first, each step of the way.

Lots of things we loved as children make great grown-up exercises, too. Thought about jumping rope lately? Well, go to the five-and-dime or just cut a length of clothesline and you're back in business. (To make sure the rope is long enough, stand on the center of it and raise each end to an armpit. If it's any shorter, you may trip yourself.) I suspect you'll find jumping a bit strenuous at first, but it's an activity that gives great return on investment. Experts estimate that ten minutes of continuous jumping equals about thirty minutes of running!

Was your last bicycle a shiny red Schwinn you got in eighth grade? Even if it's not Christmas, you might think about buying yourself a brand-new, adult-sized bike. Bicycling's good for cardiovascular fitness and builds endurance as well as muscle.

But before you take off, it's important that this bike "fit" you. Sit on the seat with your toes touching the pedals. Do your knees have a slight bend to them? If the answer is no, adjust the seat height. Your handlebars should be positioned so you're leaning only slightly forward; the dramatic almost-horizontal posture of bicycle racers isn't one to strive for as an amateur.

Having warmed up your muscles, especially the calves, you're ready. The ideal ride would include five or ten minutes across flat land, twenty minutes through some hills and then a few more minutes on flat land to cool down. (If you can't find any hills nearby, you could substitute twenty minutes of pedaling in a lower gear or riding faster.)

If you were one of those kids constantly streaking around on a pair of roller skates, you might investigate the healthful joys of contemporary skating. Apparently, today's plastic wheels make street skating a breeze, and we've all seen the exciting things that can be accomplished in the name of roller disco, on the street or indoors. But Mother's warning still holds. If you're going outside, stay well clear of any traffic.

Weight training, which encompasses weight lifting and bodybuilding, is an efficient way to increase your strength and muscle tone. But it's also something many women are turned off to initially because they think they'll end up with bulging muscles. That's not necessarily so. The key to weight training is understanding that the use of light weights with many repetitions makes for lean muscle and increased stamina. It's heavy weights with few repetitions that build bulk and strength.

Swimming has won most expert accolades for being the best all-around exercise. It engages all of your body's muscle groups, and unlike tennis or running or other sports, swimming isn't weight-bearing, so there's much less strain on your joints, much less chance of injury. But to get optimum cardiovascular benefits from swimming, you should keep going—laps or whatever—steadily, for fifteen to twenty minutes. Just splashing around with the kids doesn't count.

Then, of course, there's always an exercise class. If you're the kind that needs a group to get motivated, this could be the answer. And, as you know, when you can't make it to class, there's often the option

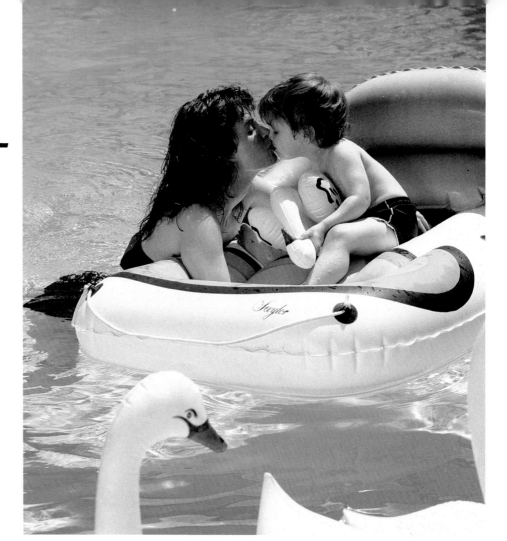

of an audio or an audiovisual cassette that allows you to go through
your paces at home.

I'm lucky enough to have my exercise "class" completely customized. The legendary Mike Abrums has developed for me (as he does
for each of his private clients) a highly individualized program, based
on posture and working the body's weaker muscle groups, for allover
fitness. The amazing thing is that his regimen is designed to take only
about fifteen or twenty minutes a day—something a person with my
sort of schedule can really appreciate.

My specific routine focuses on the muscles of my upper back and
torso, the ones that absorb all the stress, while maintaining the
strength I've always had in my spine and legs. The critical thing is to
do it *every* day.

All right, you say. I know it's important. But I don't have the time
or the money to devote to a regular, organized fitness plan. That's no
excuse. Read on.

AT-HOME FITNESS HABITS

I'm busy. You're busy. Who isn't, in today's world? But even that shouldn't tempt you to forego the energy boost and real beauty that can result from being in good shape. You can convert many of your normal, routine activities into fitness moments, with a little body awareness.

- Take a walk while you're waiting for your clothes to dry, or for the kids to get finished at the dentist's office.

- Sweep, vacuum and mop the floor with real vigor. Exaggerate those bending and stretching motions.

- Contract and release your stomach muscles, then your buttocks, while doing the dishes. This'll help alleviate any lower back pain, too.

- Elongate your spine by doing toe-touching stretches while blow-drying the underside of your hair.

- Use the stairs instead of the elevator.

- Carry the groceries in from the car one bag at a time.

- Tackle some real hills when you're taking the baby out in the stroller.

- Go disco dancing with your husband or boyfriend—and keep moving your legs, body and arms!

- When you're hanging clothes to dry, hanging curtains, or dusting the top shelves of the bookcase, really reach and stretch. Feel your muscles getting long and supple.

- When you walk the dog, *really* walk the dog! Walk briskly—about one hundred paces a minute for twenty minutes and you've covered a mile! And in an hour, you could burn 250 to 350 calories. When your canine friend stops to smell the flowers, just keep walking in place.

- If yours is a sedentary office job, try a quick walk around the block at coffee-break time. And sample these simple exercises to refresh you and wake up those bored muscles!

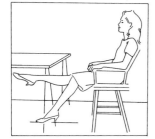

1. Push your chair back from the desk and straighten your legs, keeping the heels in contact with the floor. Point your toes and lift your right leg. Then your left. Keep alternating as you repeat.

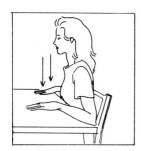

2. Now, pull your chair close to the desk. Sit up straight and suck in your stomach. Put the palms of your hands flat on the top of the desk and push down. Relax, then push again. You're not trying to lift your body's weight here. Just getting a little strengthening activity going in your shoulders and arms. Repeat.

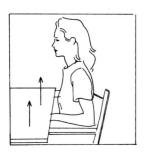

3. Next, put your hands under the edge of the desk, palms facing upward. Lift up against the weight of the desk, then release and repeat. Unless you're Wonder Woman, you don't have to worry about flipping the whole thing over!

EXERCISE: DROPPING OUT/DROPPING IN

Did you take up racquetball in all earnestness last fall, and yet couldn't begin to locate your racquet now? Have you paid your three-month, introductory membership fee at the health club and gone to its aerobics class regularly—twice? If this sounds like you, you're an exercise dropout.

You hate jogging and can't stand calisthenics? Fine. Don't do them. Dance or play tennis or take long walks with a friend. You don't really enjoy competitive sports? That's all right. Try yoga or swimming instead. Your friends all think aerobic dance class is wonderful,

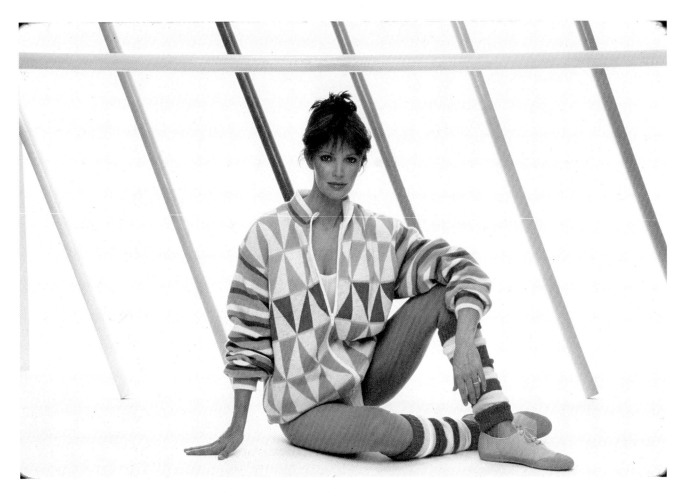

but you don't? Fair enough. Maybe you'll do better with solo activities like jogging or weight training.

I trust I've made my point. Exercise can't be a chore. It *can* be great fun and truly satisfying.

In the words of the famous commercial: "You deserve a break today." Don't try to be a drill sergeant for yourself. Take a day off from your fitness workout now and then, or change the time of day you do it. Just don't get carried away. A day or two missed won't hurt. But more than three days in a row and your fitness gains will begin to decline. You begin to lose cardiovascular fitness and your muscles start to weaken.

Ultimately, you must do your conditioning routine at least two times a week to stay in good shape. (Getting there usually takes more frequent effort.) Backsliding decreases benefits almost immediately. In just one week without exercise, the energy cells in your muscles will be reduced to half the number your conditioned muscles had. In four weeks' time, your aerobic conditioning will fall more than 17 percent.

So take a vacation from exercise if you want. But remember that two weeks missed means it'll take at least two weeks to resume the good shape you'd achieved.

VANITY VERSUS SANITY

Sure, having an attractive figure is a wonderful reason to get into a regular, enjoyable pattern of exercise. But America's fitness boom has spawned a new breed I call fitness bores. These are women and men who become obsessive, self-involved, even narcissistic. All they can talk about is their progress in weight training or how many miles they've run that week. Fitness is clearly important. An active body *does* make for an active mind, which keeps you young in form and spirit. But it's still only *one* aspect of your life. Don't sacrifice friends and family and all other interests to fitness. It's not necessary, and it's no fun!

CONVERSATION WITH AN EXPERT: MICHAEL ABRUMS ON A KNOCKOUT BODY

Michael Abrums has been developing and teaching his own unique brand of fitness for over forty-five years to a roster of clients that reads like a who's who of Hollywood stars. Mike, a kinesiologist, explains that his work is based on the study of anatomy in relation to human movement. His fitness training expertise has yielded a consistent word-of-mouth clientele, including a standing three-hundred-person waiting list. About four years ago, the name Jaclyn Smith appeared on that list; about two years ago, we began working together. Here, I ask Mike to share some of his fascinating approaches to achieving and maintaining a healthy body, and a fabulous-looking figure.

JS: As I know only too well, your first meeting with a student involves testing. Can you explain what you're looking for in those tests?

MA: Well, Jackie, the human skeleton can do nothing on its own. It's the muscles that make it move, or prevent it from moving as in the

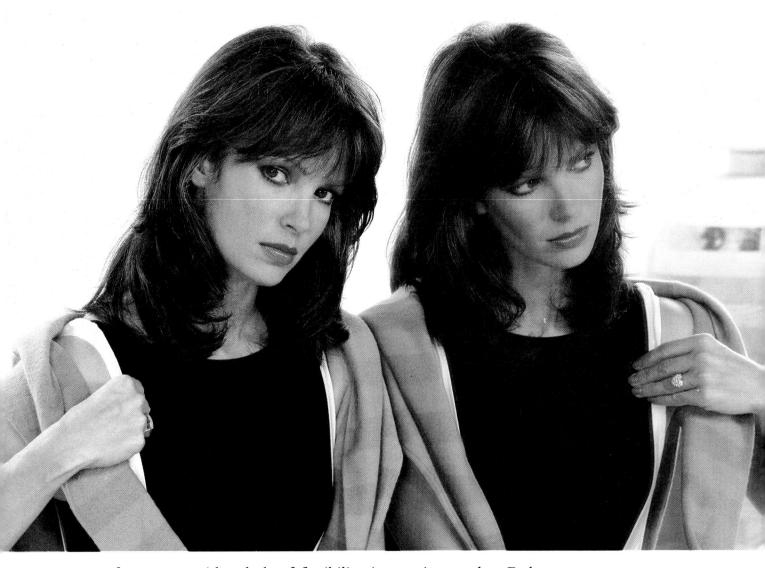

case of someone with a lack of flexibility in certain muscles. Bad posture is also often a result of muscular imbalance. For each new student, I do a posture check and then check the muscles for flexibility and strength to find out where the imbalances are. I can then create a program designed specifically for the student, where each exercise achieves a purpose without a lot of unnecessary movements.

JS: Can you describe your basic, three-phase approach to improving the body?

MA: After the posture check and review of the muscle tests, I arrive at an understanding of each individual's needs. I then work out a program which includes stretching where there is tightness, so the body is able to assume the correct position, and I begin strengthening the muscles that pull the body back and hold it in the correct position. When a female student is first able to assume this new position, she feels like the bride of Frankenstein's monster—if a man, like the monster itself. So the third part is to reeducate the proprioceptive senses to the fact that the new position is the right one. I do this by showing the student various ways to teach her body to assume the correct position throughout the day till that position begins to feel normal and easy.

JS: One of the most amazing things about your approach, Mike, and one of the things that make it so appealing to me, is that you believe in spending only about fifteen minutes a day on this. And yet you get such great results. Just how do you do it?

MA: There are so many myths surrounding this whole question of bodily fitness, not the least of which is "no sweat, no pain, no gain." Let me explain why that is simply not accurate. Working out for one or two hours and sweating profusely is not necessary for fitness. Perspiring has nothing to do with fitness. The purpose of your sudoriferous glands is to lower body temperature, not to lose fat. A lot of people feel that if they are not sweating buckets, they are not getting a workout. Perspiring doesn't even represent any real weight loss. If you happen to perspire a lot, sure you'll lose some weight. But drink a glass of water and you're right back where you started. Reducing calorie intake and increasing output is the best way to lose weight. So, the woman who sweats more than another in a gym class isn't necessarily getting more fit, she is simply sweating more. Furthermore, the practice of wearing rubber sweat suits, body wraps, and so on should be avoided, because it can lead to problems and is of no benefit.

On to the question of pain. It's a shame so many people are knocking themselves out doing multi-repetition exercises that don't have any effect on the area they think they're working. If a certain muscle hurts while exercising, they assume they're working that area. Not necessarily so. As an example: one of my students asked for and received permission to bring in a friend of hers visiting from New York. During the session, the friend asked me why, when she was doing two hundred repetitions a day of the raised-leg-out-to-the-side exercise, she still had flabby inner thighs. She said, "My inner thighs

(opposite): *Tennis—or any sport you love to do— is a great fitness choice. As you can see, my real skill here is in refereeing.*

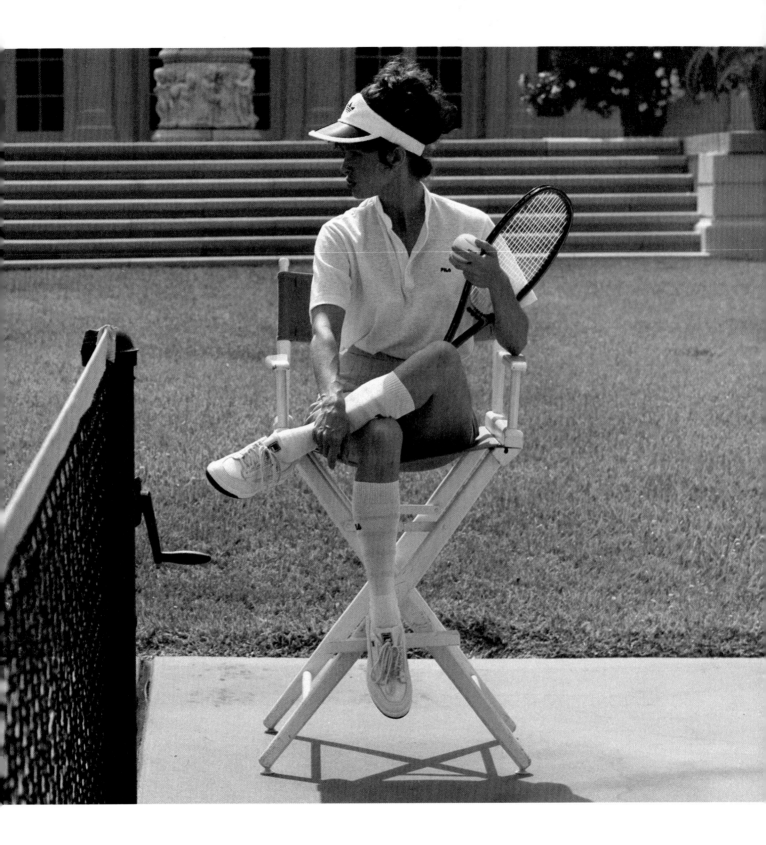

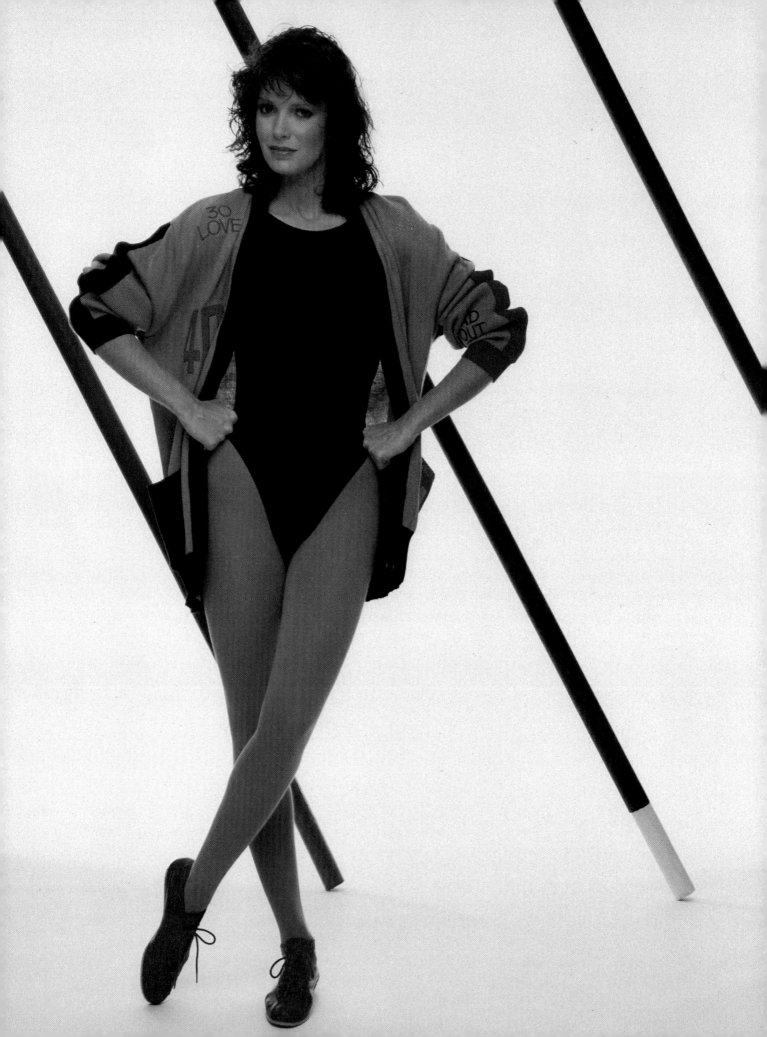

hurt like the dickens whenever I do that exercise, so I must be working that muscle, but I still get no results." Before answering her, I tested the flexibility of her leg adductors (the inner thigh muscles) and, as I expected, they were very tight. I explained to her that in reality she was working the leg abductors—the muscle that brought the leg out to the side—and that the reason for the pain was the tightness in her inner thigh muscles. Here was a case of pain, but no gain.

If people, especially the teachers, were more knowledgeable about the physiological action of the muscles, workouts would become shorter. It simply isn't necessary to suffer during exercises. Muscles may be toned and fitness obtained without exhausting oneself. Because the body deconditions itself so rapidly, exercise must be regular, but it's not realistic to assume that one can exercise regularly for one to two hours a day as long as a person lives. Most people don't have the energy, time, or desire to face that. But it is realistic to assume that one could and would exercise fifteen minutes a day for the rest of one's life.

JS: What about weight loss?

MA: Just as my program is realistic in terms of exercise—fifteen minutes a day is a truly feasible lifelong plan for maintaining your body, wouldn't you say?—well, that's my approach to diet, too. I give most of my pupils a custom diet plan. In general, my ideas are based upon anything in moderation. I believe in eating natural foods as much as possible: turkey, fish, chicken, some eggs, no salts or sugar, a minimum of fats, lots of vegetables, salads, some fruit and whole grains. Nothing earth-shatteringly new. It's unrealistic— there's that word again—and frankly depressing to think of life stretching before you with a denial of everything "bad," with ice cream or cake never entering the picture again. I say, eat a little of your favorite junk food, if you must, but adjust for it the next day. However, it must be understood that when you are trying to reach your "fighting weight," the results would be much quicker if you abstained from these foods entirely.

JS: Your customized programs always involve work with weights. Aren't some of your female clients wary of looking like weight lifters?

MA: Some may be initially. But they quickly learn that, first, resistance movements develop the muscles fastest, and second, that I'm a firm believer in a woman's developing a little muscle definition without ever becoming unfeminine. To me, that means slimness, firmness, but also roundness to the body, too. I've advocated exercise with weights through all the years of my teaching, but I've always watched very carefully to make sure that there was no overdevelopment in any area of the body. In each individual, different areas of the body develop faster than others, and if the teacher is not there all the time, some hideous results come about. Women are being told they can't develop muscles. I think you'll agree, when you see the women bodybuilders of today, that that's not true. Now, some actually prefer a high degree of muscularity in women; I do not.

JS: I suppose the very best way to illustrate how your unique system works would be to share some of the exercises you've worked out for me, but please don't embarrass me too much.

MA: No need to, Jackie. Remember when we started working together, one of your problems was abducted scapula; that is, your "wings" were protruding in the back, which caused you to appear round-shouldered. As I explained, this postural deviation was caused by a muscular imbalance: your pectoral (chest) muscles were too tight, and your scapular adductors—the muscles in your upper back—were underdeveloped. We worked on several things to stretch the pecs, as when I had you sit on a narrow bench, with your fingers touching behind your head, and I very gently pulled your elbows back and up. When you are not with me, you are to lie on the floor with your knees bent, feet on the floor, a pillow doubled up behind your shoulders, the top part of the pillow even with your shoulders. In this position, you put your hands behind your head, fingers touching, and allow your head and elbows to fall back, the weight of your head and arms gently stretching the pectorals (and if necessary, press the elbows down to the floor gently).

At the same time, to strengthen the adductors, I started you out by doing this exercise: while sitting, elbows bent so fingertips meet in front of nose (palms down), do the pelvic tilt. That is, squeeze the buttocks and hold throughout the exercise. Rotating palms forward, touch fingertips together behind your head. Elbows lead the motion; do not move your head; keep fingers extended. As you well know, we advanced to exercises with a greater degree of difficulty to further strengthen those muscles. As you became stronger, the difficulty of the exercises increased.

JS: With so many of your students in show business, you often have us send you videotapes of our work on television or in films. Why is that?

MA: Well, that's the only way I can check whether a student has really been reeducated to carry him or herself correctly. When I'm with a student, he or she is conscious of what we've learned about posture. It's when they are away from me that I can see how much they've really absorbed—it's also a way to check how well they are maintaining their weight. I have to laugh on those occasions when I attend a party full of my students. The moment I walk in, there is an instant shift around the room, as they assume their correct postures. But the real goal of my work with my students is to make that correct carriage, with proper muscular support, a natural part of their lives. That's the only way to have a fabulous body—for life.

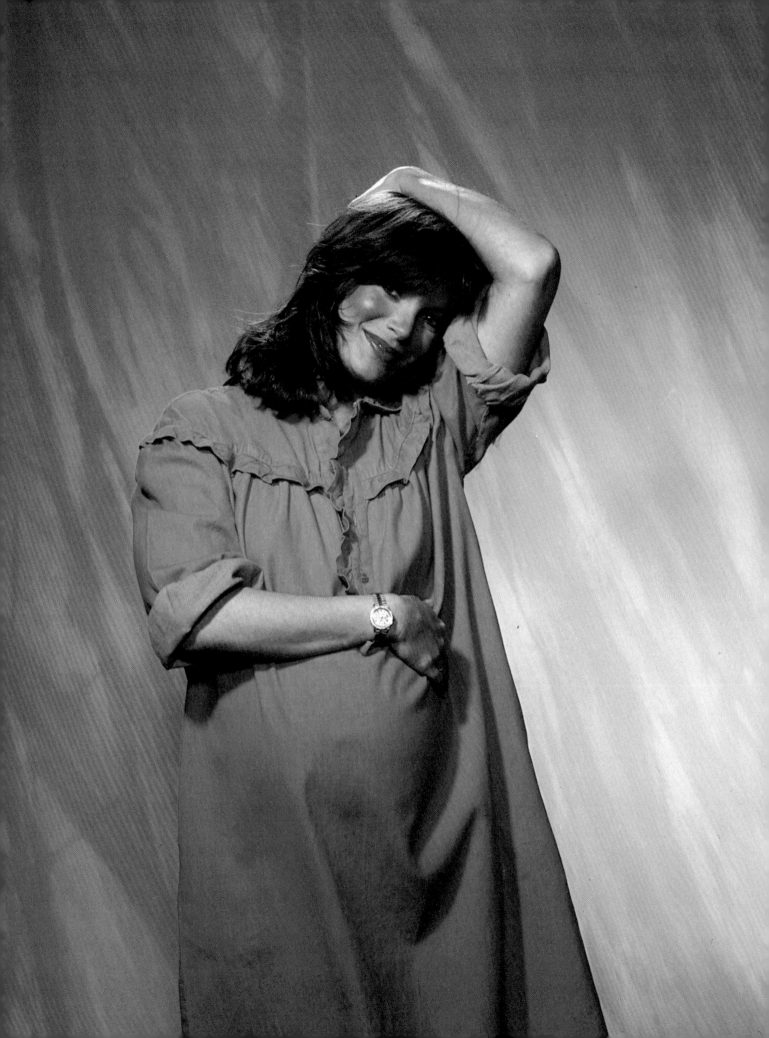

CHAPTER 9

So You're Going to Have a Baby?

People may say it's not a unique experience, but I so clearly remember feeling I was the most special woman on earth when I learned I was pregnant with Gaston, my nearly three-year-old son. Since I was no longer in my twenties when Tony and I were married, and since I had at other times in my life been on birth-control pills, I had no reason to expect to become pregnant right away. But I did! It was only within two months of my first visit to my gynecologist to discuss the fact that Tony and I wanted a child.

Just about a month and a half after that visit, I began feeling a bit tired and slightly nauseated, which was highly unusual for me. My internist agreed that pregnancy was unlikely, so she ran tests for other possible explanations—influenza or anemia or something like that. Finally, I suggested we include the pregnancy test and sure enough, the results were positive.

The timing for my pregnancy was perfect in so many regards. I had just finished shooting "Jacqueline Bouvier Kennedy" and had already decided to wait for another equally challenging role. That one was so

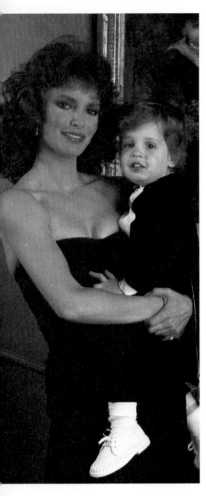

With my son, Gaston, who made me realize that being a mother is the most important, satisfying role I'll ever play

special, such a departure for me that I wanted time to absorb the public's reaction, too. So I had no immediate plans for work, except for some commercials and still photographs for Max Factor.

That commitment wasn't a problem for me because, except for some fullness in my face and a little water retention in my ankles and hands, my pregnancy really wasn't obvious until the sixth month. I hoped they could use contouring to bring my face down a bit, to get a Jaclyn Smith look consistent with all the other ads. It was funny, though, that the bright side of my facial fullness was endless compliments about how young I looked!

I began taking prenatal vitamins daily, right away. I credit them with the almost instant change in my fingernails and hair. My nails, which normally verge on the paper-thin, became so strong. And my always-thick hair became even more beautifully thick and lustrous. My skin, too, had a marvelously smooth texture and wonderful natural color. In fact, I'd say that that was my complexion's finest hour.

I do realize how lucky I was in all this; I know it isn't always the same for every woman. I didn't even get stretch marks! I rubbed my skin with vitamin-E oil every night and found that after it was all over and I'd regained my normal weight, I had less evidence of marks than many women who've not been pregnant at all but have merely developed stretch marks in the course of losing and gaining significant weight.

My pregnancy was such an overwhelmingly positive experience, even though I do remember having a bit of nausea at times in the first trimester. And my energy level, as I mentioned, wasn't up to par, so I do have mental images of myself crawling into bed at eight o'clock some nights, not feeling all that terrific.

Also, during those first three months, I was plagued with very serious headaches. My doctor explained that I was feeling all the expanding that was going on in my body as pressure, that is, headaches. Since I refused to take so much as an aspirin during my pregnancy, I found relief in the form of pressure-point massage.

A masseuse would come to my house and sometimes concentrate her efforts on my head for as much as an hour, with just a little extra time devoted to massaging those points on my feet that, according to the masseuse, corresponded to my pain. All I know is that if I got into bed for the night immediately following the massage, I could count on waking up headache-free the next morning. She was my lifesaver!

I still often indulge in pressure-point massages, considering them a necessary luxury. And since I'm always so pressed for time, guaranteed results are important. That experience during my pregnancy brought me to the conviction that pressure-point massage—precisely because it is more focused—is preferable to standard Swedish massage for tension reduction and muscle relaxation.

During my second trimester, my only slight problem was with occasional pressure against my rib cage. When struck with one of these pains, I'd stretch out on a bed or sofa to find relief. Not a big deal, especially considering that I was completely spared the constant back pain so many women experience.

The third trimester was the best I felt: no nausea, no headaches, no pain in the ribs. I could simply enjoy the expectation of my baby.

KEEPING UP A FASHIONABLE FRONT

At first, since I wasn't so big, clothes didn't present much of a problem. I could find fashionable skirts and blouses like the Ralph Lauren prairie-look clothes that were in then as well as corduroys that could be elasticized to grow with me. To go with my pants—I also had a faithful pair of jeans with the elastic front panel—I didn't buy maternity tops; I'd simply buy oversized shirts and sweaters. Tony got used to my raiding his closets for these items, too.

But then I got to the point where the two-piece approach wasn't working for me anymore. I needed a one-piece, clean-lined silhouette to make me look neat and as small as possible. Even so, the dresses I bought or had made were no-waisted styles, a couple of sizes larger than normal, not specially designed for expectant mothers. I was very disappointed that it was so difficult to find maternity clothes that were sophisticated and well made. After all, the fact that you're pregnant doesn't mean you've instantly fallen in love with polyester or billowing smock tops with pert bows under the chin.

As I got larger and larger in the middle, I concentrated on accessories that would make me feel truly pretty and feminine. Lovely shoes, jewelry and, as was the vogue then, lots of lace stockings. Plus, for evening wear, there was one Yves Saint Laurent dress, a tent-shaped chemise all in black velvet and taffeta ruffles, that made me feel spectacular. The point is it's worth the effort to wear truly nice things because these are nine months when a woman really wants to look happy and pretty.

That reminds me of the whole episode of the *Time* magazine cover of me, pregnant. For a story on the baby-boom generation becoming parents, having children in their thirties, the editors asked if I'd give an interview about my own experience and pose for a cover shot. I

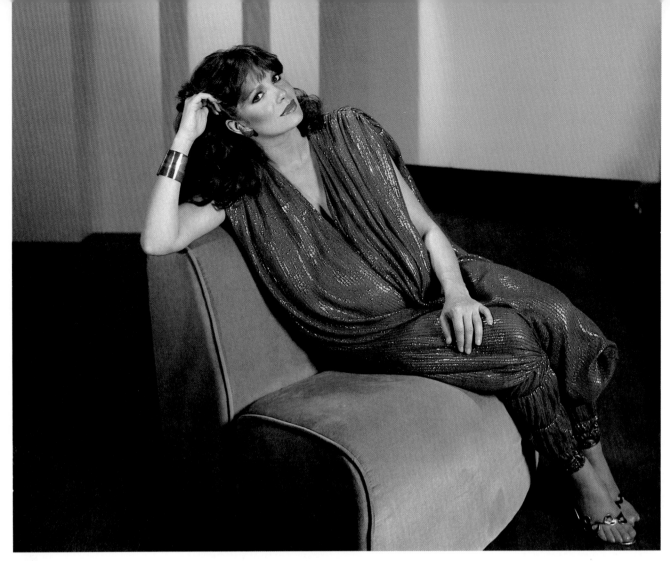

agreed, and we did an initial photo session with me wearing a fabulous, shimmery Norma Kamali jumpsuit. (It was the sort of thing a "normal" woman would have worn belted, but I wore it loose.) I thought the whole thing looked great, and fun, but for some reason, the editors didn't like the results.

So, we decided to shoot another cover-try (as they're called in the business), with me in my own blue denim jumper this time. That's the picture America saw—shot from underneath. Boy, did I look pregnant! And what a complete contrast to my tight-pants, Charlie's Angels image!

I was disappointed in that shot, not because of vanity, but because it didn't catch the sense of exuberance, the through-and-through happiness I was feeling. I wanted that photo to be, literally, full of life.

I've kept a copy of that issue, of course, and think that when he's old enough to look at it, Gaston will get a kick out of the fact that he and I were on the cover of *Time* magazine together!

EATING FOR TWO

Even though throughout my first trimester, on-again, off-again nausea pretty much killed my appetite, *nothing* interfered with my breakfast! I ate pancakes, eggs, bacon, toast, you name it. And Tony fixed us both healthful, delicious dinners. He even discovered a special treat he could make for me. He put a lot of fresh fruit in the blender—coconut, papaya, banana—and then froze the results into a wonderful, frosty drink. I loved those at night; they were my "chocolate cake."

Otherwise, I found myself eating the recommended crackers and plain breads to absorb some of the acidity in my system, and then, just plain, good food: celery, carrots, other vegetables and fruits and just a minimum of meat and fish.

My appetite picked up in my fourth month, and I really began eating three square meals a day, sometimes with snacks in between. I don't think I overate, because being too full is a genuinely uncomfortable experience when you're pregnant. On the other hand, I had decided not to worry about gaining weight. I wanted to enjoy this time as much as possible, and so ate exactly what I wanted, when I wanted.

You always hear of expectant mothers developing unusual cravings, and mine was particularly appalling to Tony. I became absolutely mad for fast-food hamburgers—and there was my gourmet husband, who thought I was completely insane. He doesn't even consider hamburgers food!

All in all, I managed to gain forty pounds, and, though my doctor assured me that it wasn't excessive, there were fleeting moments when I couldn't picture myself thin again. But overriding all such concerns was the fact that I wanted this little baby more than anything.

SPECIAL DELIVERY

Here's the scene: I was three days past my due date, and a bit nervous that Tony was shooting a film that often kept him at work until eleven or twelve at night. When I woke up that morning, I had felt different, with a slight sense of pain, or pressure, really. As the afternoon approached, that sensation continued, but I thought it didn't hurt enough to be "the real thing." My mother, who was staying with us, felt we should time the contractions, and as we discovered they were coming about every five minutes, we called the doctor. He arrived at the house in the early evening and noted that I was already five centi-

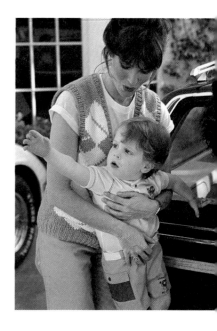

meters dilated. (Ten centimeters is considered optimum for giving birth.) I had been resting all day—my mother and my trusted assistant wouldn't even let me wash my hair—so I was perfectly ready to go on to the hospital at about six-thirty that evening.

As serious labor came upon me, I used all the pain-relieving and mind-diverting techniques I'd learned at Lamaze class. I was truly able to "be there," to bear the pain without any muscle relaxants or other drugs. I know it may sound unbelievable, but I enjoyed every second of it.

Tony made it to the hospital from his film set in time to help with the final pushing. He was so proud of me, and I was so happy he was there. Finally, at 12:33 A.M. on March 19, 1982, we met our son, Gaston.

I already knew his name, you see, because Tony and I had made a deal beforehand. If the baby was a little girl, he'd get to name her. If it was a boy, I would name him Gaston Anthony Richmond—Gaston after my grandfather, Anthony after my husband.

Despite our agreement, Tony and my mother did pressure me a bit to reconsider, arguing that Gaston was too unusual a name. But I'd always dreamed of having a son of my own to name after my beloved grandfather, and stood my ground. But, of course, as Gaston grows older and goes off to school, if he chooses to go by Anthony or Tony, well, that's his decision.

GETTING IT ALL TOGETHER AGAIN

I was back home from the hospital in four or five days, still rather tired, but very excited. However, since the last thing on my mind was going out to buy a whole new wardrobe, I did immediately turn my attention to getting back into shape, so I could fit into my clothes!

The birth itself was a big boost, when it came to weight loss. At least it was in my case. I gave birth to a seven-pound-fifteen-ounce baby, and lost nearly twenty pounds in the process. You do the arithmetic!

But quite seriously, I had eschewed all exercises during the pregnancy, except for those taught in Lamaze classes, because I was just too afraid something might go wrong, especially since I wasn't exactly a 22-year-old having her first child. Nor did I start exercising right away after the birth, while I was first breast-feeding.

Breast-feeding, however, did present a rather compelling reason to watch very carefully that everything I consumed was pure and whole-

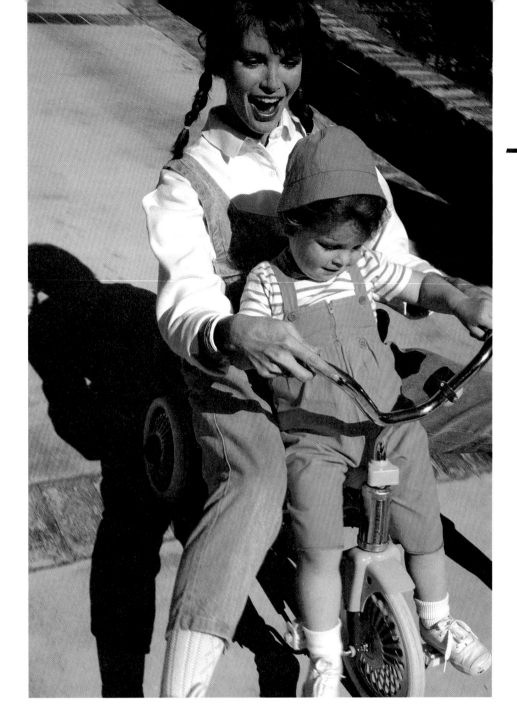

some. I drank no soft drinks, ate no chocolate, made sure my Chinese food was free of monosodium glutamate. All to be on the very safe side.

I did eat vegetables, chicken, fish, some red meat, cheese and dairy products, but cut out snacking between meals. (Apparently, breast-feeding makes some women quite ravenous, but I found it made me positively un-hungry.) Never one to totally deprive myself, I indulged in Italian food from time to time.

I heartily recommend breast-feeding to all new mothers who are interested and *relaxed* about the idea. As well as being a calorie-burning activity that can help with the initial weight loss, it's a marvelously close time with your baby. I loved every intimate minute of it.

However, those minutes were cut short by, of all things, the arrival of a fabulous script. It wasn't an easy decision to make, but knowing that a role like mine in "Rage of Angels" doesn't come along all that often, I took it, even though it meant I'd have to give up breast-feeding after four months, rather than the six I had planned to devote to it. (I was much relieved to learn that the critical immunities a mother passes along through breast-feeding are achieved after the third month.)

With that role to prepare for, I really had to gear up on my route back to a thin, taut body. I began exercising with Mike Abrums again in his concentrated fifteen-minute sessions six days a week. And as the first shooting date on "Rage" approached, I honed my meals down to the true, healthy essentials: chicken, vegetables, salads and fish, with red meat included only if it was very lean. Plus, I often did an extra fifteen minutes of my Abrums workout at night, before going to bed. I became as strict as I've ever been—had to be!—with myself. And of course, time with my husband and baby was just as important. But I was willing and able to discipline myself because it was so clearly worth it. *Everything* in my life was perfect—my child, my marriage, my career. Ultimately, it took me only two months total to make it back to my ideal weight of about 115 pounds.

It is a time of my life I look back on with a sense of wonder. I was amazed at how all the elements of my life seemed to come together at

Gaston and I stop for a hug before taking the dogs for a walk.

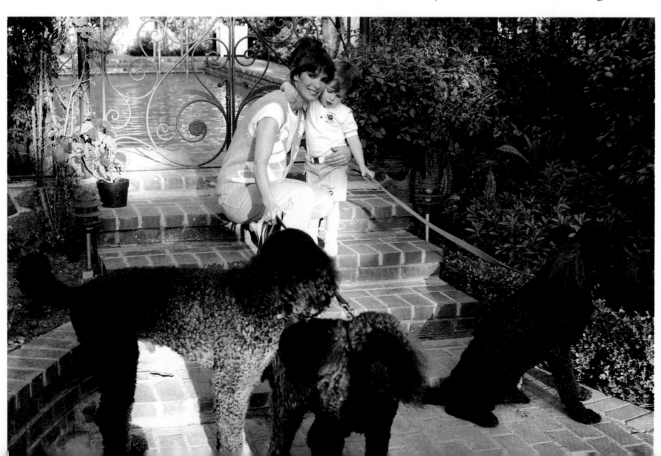

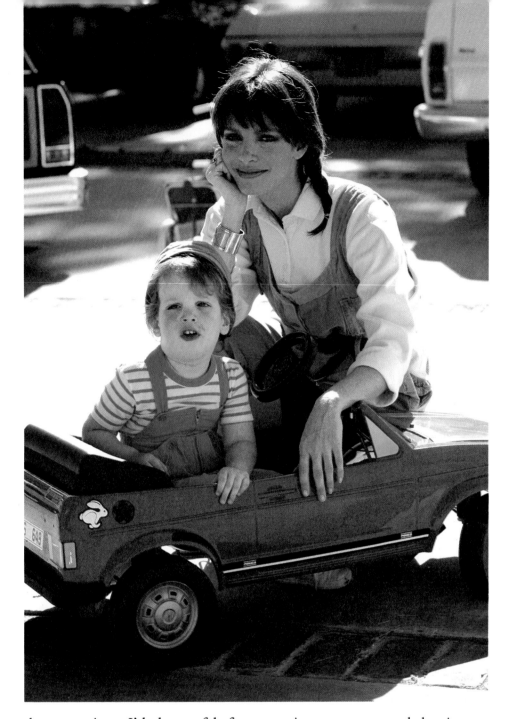

the same time. I'd always felt fortunate in my career, and that it was going forward in the direction I'd planned, but there was always a nagging sense of something missing. A child. So when I look at Gaston and say he's adorable, he's brilliant, he's a miracle, that's all understatement for me.

And believe me, I hope I never forget that wonderful peace, that calm—and I'm a worrier by nature!—that swept over me for those nine months before Gaston came into my life.

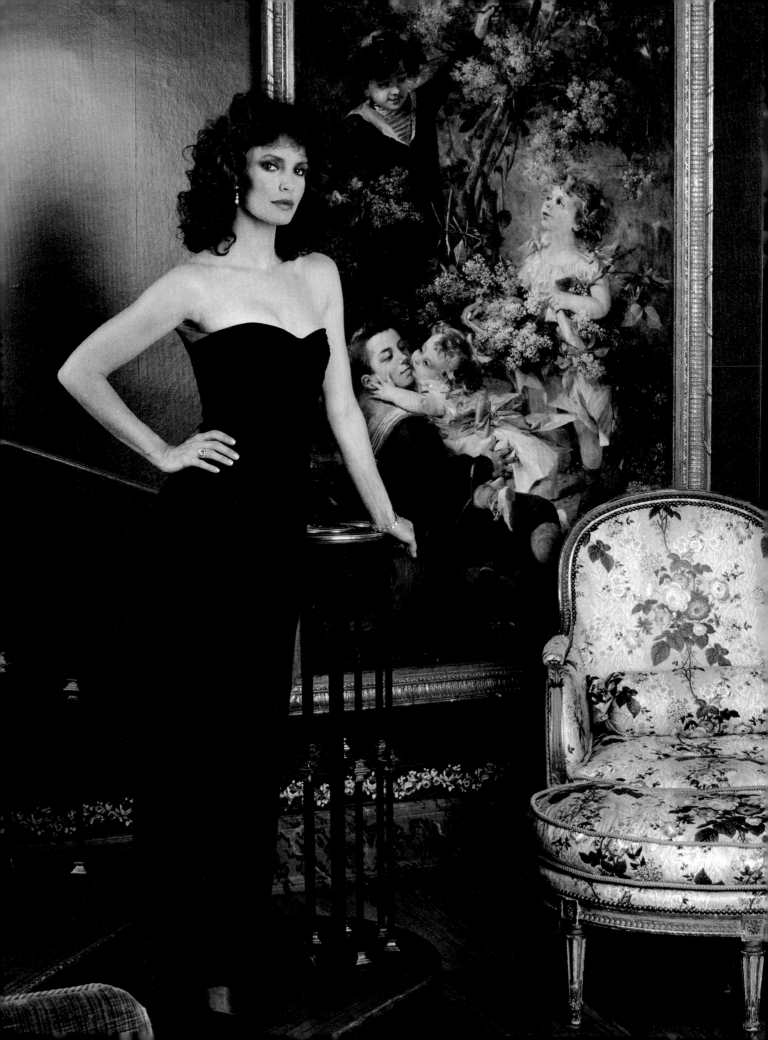

CHAPTER 10

Your Body: Care and Clothing

When you think about it, your body is so many things. It's skin you want always to be smooth and attractively soft; it's all those marvelous muscles and tendons and ligaments you want toned and yet supple; it's a tall or short, lean or round "package" that has so much to do with the image others have of you as well as your own self-image. And not least of all, its outer wrapping—the clothes you choose to put on it—sends clear and immediate messages about just who you think you are. Clearly, bearing all this responsibility in life, your body deserves your attention.

IN MOVEMENT

We've talked at some length about exercise in chapter 8, both structured and informal ways to get muscle-toning and fitness benefits. But there's an additional point I'd like to make. I think many of us make the mistake of thinking of exercise *only* in terms of losing weight, or maintaining an attractive, appealing figure. Both are great

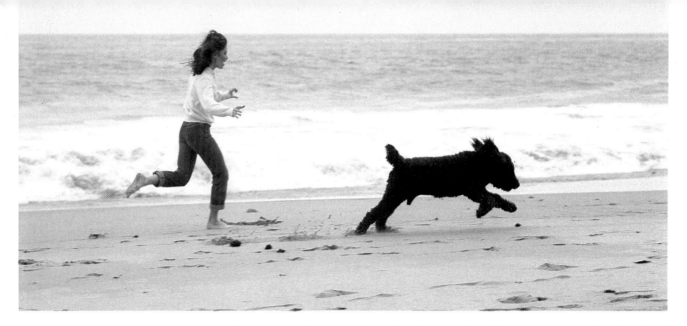

motivators, to be sure. But there's another factor to consider. Each of us is going to get older, inevitably. And I, for one, want to be as active as possible all my life.

So, beyond being trim, there's the vision of being fit and mobile, in the most basic sense, when I'm older. And that goal requires, I think, a long-term approach to exercise, sports, body movement, whatever you want to call it. Regardless of how thin or shapely one is, keeping the body fluid, loose and active is a day-in, day-out investment of effort, starting now. You can never give up on it, and why should you? I guess what I'm asking, simply put, is do you see yourself playing nine holes of golf when you're sixty-five, seventy, seventy-five? Or do you prefer the vision of literally sitting out the last ten years of your life? What you do now—the fitness habits you develop—can make all the difference.

MASSAGE

I'm a great believer in the benefits of massage, especially pressure-point (often called Shiatsu) massage, which I first discovered as a magnificent headache reducer during my pregnancy. The more common Swedish massage is also a marvelous way to loosen tightened muscles and reduce some of the bodily manifestations of stress.

I am fortunate to have a talented masseuse (in fact, I've *never* had a masseur massage me) who comes regularly to my home. And, in all truth, I think both Shiatsu and Swedish massage are impossible to perform successfully on oneself. Of course, there's always the attractive option of switching off with the man in your life, when it comes to home-administered massages. But I would recommend that at least

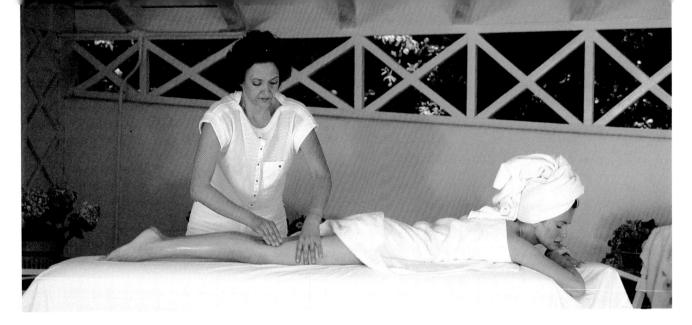

one of you see a professional Swedish-style masseuse or masseur first, to get some good moves down. Also, use some kind of lubricant— baby oil, your body lotion, or whatever—when giving an amateur massage.

There is, however, one aspect of Shiatsu massage that can lend itself to self-administration. It's a sort of subspecialty of pressure-point massage dealing with mapped-out points on the feet that are believed to correspond to all the organs and muscle groups in the body. If you're interested, I suggest the library, where books on Oriental massage techniques, or more specifically, on reflexology are sure to be obtainable.

European women have long believed in the benefits—most often described as anticellulite action—of self-massage. And there are several massage-mitt-and-cream kits available now in the United States. I certainly don't think there's any harm in combining some aspect of self-massage with the bathing ritual. But I can't comment on these cellulite systems because, thank God, I don't have any cellulite to work on—at least, not yet. (I think my dancer's training has spared me that beauty problem.)

Even untrained massage of your own feet during a hot bath, or simple toward-the-heart massage of the legs and torso while you're applying body lotion, can be a relaxing and soothing experience. So why not?

MAKE MINE SMOOTH

Having allover smooth skin is the result of a combination of factors: moisture, sun exposure and hair removal.

Obviously, the parts of your body most frequently exposed to sun, cold air, wind, heat, pollution, etc., need greater attention than the usually covered parts. That's why the neck, chest and hands warrant conscientious moisturizing and sunscreening; the elbows and hidden-but-hardworking feet, regular pumicing or sloughing. As for the rest of your body, the rather simple-to-attain habit of smoothing on a fast-absorbing body lotion after every shower or bath should keep these unexposed areas soft.

You may notice some changes, however, after a holiday or summer season that has involved a lot of running around in the sun in a bikini or other body-baring garb. Some women experience recurring discolorations or simple freckling of the skin on their stomachs, lower backs or lower chests, revealed by a décolleté swimsuit. These discolorations, even when they occur on more-often-exposed legs and arms, signal a site of hyperpigmentation or hypopigmentation in the skin cells, and normally fade during the winter months. I have nothing against freckles; a few sprinkled across the nose can be positively charming. But if you're not keen on encouraging body freckles, the only answer is careful use of a total sunblock.

Dangerous discolorations are those that continue to change, darken or enlarge, with or without continued exposure to sunlight. They may signal anything from a nonmalignant mole to a keratosis. In any case, it's time to consult your dermatologist.

The options on hair removal are many, and finding the right one for you is most often a process of trial and, unfortunately, error. Underarms are easily shaved in your daily shower or bath, though some women do have their underarms waxed—ouch!—preferring the longer-lasting results and the relatively sparse regrowth promised with waxing. (The only difficulty being that waxing is most efficient when performed on several days' growth.)

Legs, too, are easily shaved, daily, or can be waxed. Although it necessarily involves some degree of pain, I happen to prefer waxing for my lower legs and always have a professional do it for me. I've tried waxing my legs myself but have found that you have to whip those wax-coated linen strips off at a certain angle to get really smooth results. A salon job almost always guarantees a little savings in pain. I think it's worth it!

There are also, of course, many foam and cream depilatories on the market. The only caution here, as mentioned on the packaging, is to test the product on your skin to be certain you don't get a reaction. If there's lasting redness or a rash after use, it's probably not the product for you.

Both at-home depilatories and salon waxing can take care of other unwanted body hair—the bikini line, hair on the stomach or breasts. But when it's a question of facial hair, electrolysis and bleaching head the list of possibilities. (Needless to say, shaving is *never* the answer when dealing with facial hair.)

I've not had any firsthand experience with these techniques, but friends and acquaintances have said that electrolysis and bleaching are effective methods for coping with unwanted facial hair. It seems to me that bleaching would be the less frightening, not to mention less painful, alternative. But many women do find aestheticians and electrolysis experts they trust and have no negative reactions to the necessarily repetitious treatments. So the choice is, as always, up to you.

THE BRONZED BODY

As I've noted, I love a touch of golden tan on my body, especially my legs. But not being a sunbather per se, I find I can pick up enough color just playing with Gaston or bicycling with Tony. And I do mean enough, even though I always wear at least some protection, say, a sunscreen of SPF 6 or greater. (SPF stands for sun protection factor, as is clearly labeled on almost all sun-care products these days.)

Since I also cover my face with a sunblock and/or a hat that shades me from almost all direct and reflected rays, there are occasions when there's a tone difference between my face and body. To even things up, I've found dusting my powder blush—a peachy apricot or a pink, or both—down on my neck and onto my chest will camouflage most

California living means pretty umbrellas and lots of sunscreen.

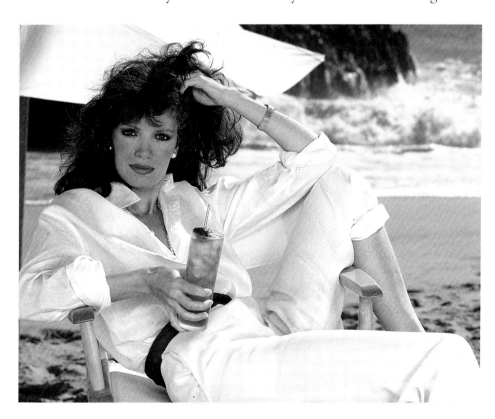

such discrepancies. If there's a more marked line of demarcation, I'll extend my foundation, mixed with water, as always, down to my neck and blend it into my chest before applying the powder blush.

One of the great boons to women who love a tan and yet are fully aware of the aging effects of the sun, is the improved no-sun tanner. Today, chemically achieved or natural, plant-extract bronzers are available that, although they necessarily stain the skin somewhat, don't leave that telltale orangy tint of yesterday's tanners. They're great for allover use (always, according to the directions) or just for filling in a strap mark or a dress neckline that plunges lower than your bathing suit.

Without any scientific evidence to go by, I'm not a big fan of tanning parlors. Even if they're not harmful to your skin, I think it's such a waste of time to sit or stand in one of those machines just to get a bit of color that can easily be achieved cosmetically.

Cosmetic bronzers, temporary, sheer-color gels, usually, are another viable way to even up the score if your body is tanner than your face.

CLOTHING YOUR BODY

Clothes are such a highly individual matter, and yet there exist, it seems to me, some generally applicable principles that go into dressing well. For example, far from being a fashion faddist myself, I do believe that change is one of the most exciting things about life. I think it's a mistake for a woman to get one, unalterable image of herself and never leave it. I mean, it's a bit sad to see a grown woman dressing like a little girl, for instance. On the other hand, no matter what her age, if a woman has fabulous legs, why shouldn't she show them off in a short, even mini, skirt if it's within the broad spectrum of fashion at the time?

One of the great joys of being a woman today is being able to indulge different moods and different self-images through clothes. Unless you're a very dramatic personality who can wear one look all the time, like Coco Chanel in her then-controversial uniform of black jersey pants and cardigans, experimentation is fun!

I think you have to make up your own mind about what suits *you*. Of course, the man in your life might have an opinion you'll want to take into consideration. But shopping with your mother or girlfriends or a man can be a very confusing experience. It's sometimes hard to decide what *you* actually think about how you look when you're

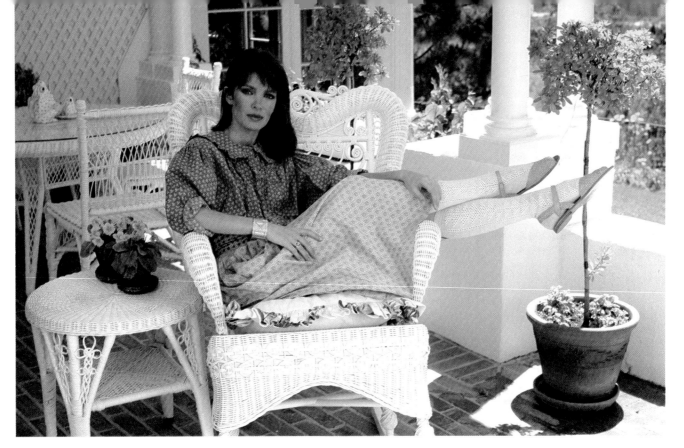

fielding others' opinions at the same time. But if you're not completely confident about your own taste, a trusted friend or even a department store's personal shopper can be of valuable assistance.

I must say, I have such limited time for shopping myself that I have to go alone and work fast. I even have some help from salespeople in Los Angeles stores who understand my taste, will call me about things they think I might like, and then send them over for me to try on.

I love clothes, well-made clothes from a variety of designers, American, French and Italian. And I love experimenting with my real-life wardrobe. Maybe that's because my television and film clothes have to be conservative. They can be contemporary but conservative enough not to look odd in the reruns.

I tend to prefer solid colors to prints and, I suppose, because of my dark hair and green eyes, wear a lot of khaki, brown, black, beige and green—dark green. I often toss in some bright colors, such as turquoise or hot pink, during the summer or when I'm in a tropical climate. And I adore white for all-year-round wear.

I'm tall enough and thin enough to carry off most silhouettes, but there are some limitations. For example, a straight-cut, midcalf-length skirt, which may be part of a very romantic twenties look, just doesn't suit me because my legs are thin. That sort of skirt seems to cut off the line at an unflattering point.

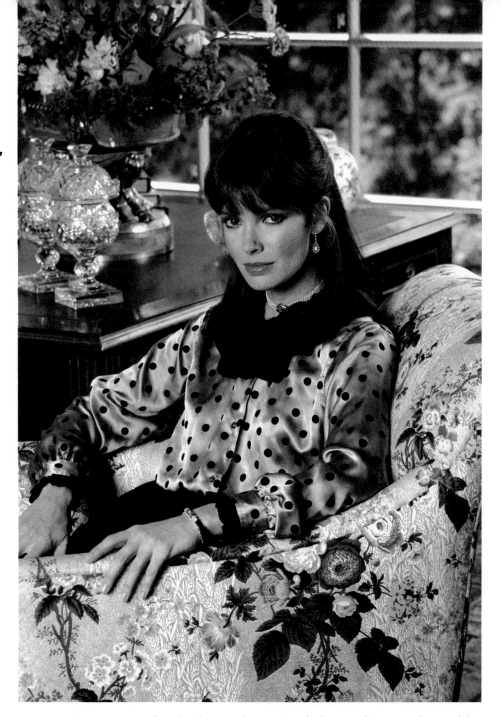

I'm also not too fond of straight-up-and-down dress styles. I like evening dresses that are more contoured to the body and day dresses that are defined at the waist. Belts, in fact, are one of my passions. I collect them in all widths, skinny to five or six inches wide, depending on the whole outfit's proportion. I have a favorite antique belt buckle I uncovered at one of the flea markets in Paris, and I plan to collect more in future travels.

Although Tony's appreciation of them has gotten me into many more skirts—above the knee if they're straight; ankle length if they're full and flowing—I haven't abandoned pants. Again, because of my thin legs, I don't think cropped-just-below-the-calf pant styles look great on me; I prefer the more narrow tailored trousers that go to the ankle whether they're pleated gray flannels or corduroys.

As far as tops are concerned, I wear everything from button-down, oxford-cloth shirts to strapless, sequined after-dark camisoles to high-collared, lacy Victorian blouses. The only neckline I object to, on me, is a too-wide scoop-neck or a boat-neck style.

If I lived in a cooler climate, I think I would really love to wear furs. As it is, I own a coyote coat that I feel is the warmest thing going. My ultimate, though, is fur-lined garments. Having the fur on the inside, with you, is the warmest, the most luxurious feeling in the world.

I like the new ultrasoft, pliant designs that are being made of leathers and suedes these days, but I wouldn't wear a complete leather outfit. It's still too reminiscent of the motorcycle moll look, for my taste. But a leather skirt or trousers? Great.

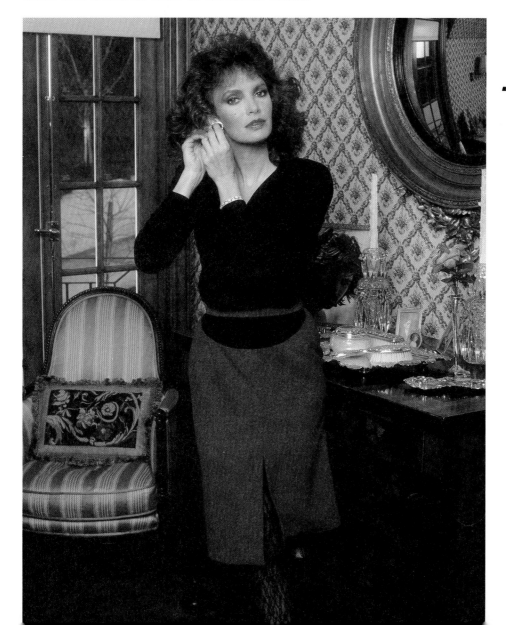

Tony's appreciation of skirts and pretty stockings has gotten me wearing them more.

169

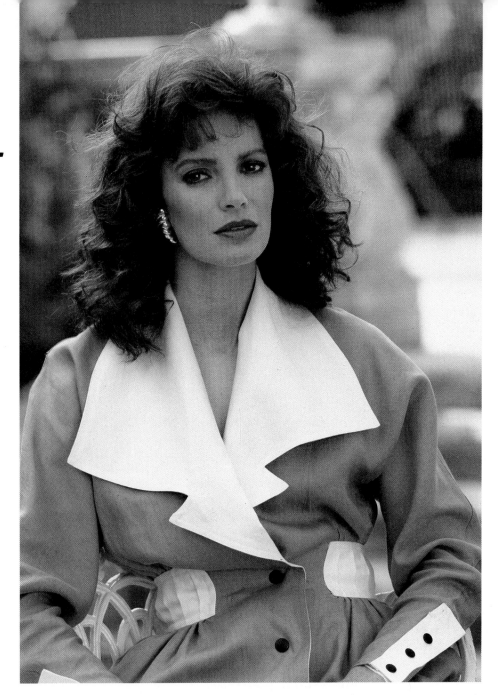

*Dramatic details—contrast
coloring, oversized collar,
decorative buttons—jazz
up a basically conservative
look.*

On the one hand, I love getting dressed up and accenting the look with jewelry. Antique jewelry is a favorite, though there are modern designs I also like. On the other hand, jumpsuits and sweats are super —comfortable and a real part of my wardrobe, too.

The biggest change in my recent life—Gaston—has produced the biggest change in my wardrobe. While pregnant, I got very used to wearing flats, ballet slippers and tennis shoes. I love the look of high heels, but I'm still in the process of reintroducing my feet to the sensation and limited movement those sexy evening shoes offer.

CONVERSATION WITH AN EXPERT: NOLAN MILLER ON STYLE

A professional costume designer for film, theater and television for nearly thirty years, Nolan Miller has dressed stars ranging from Joan Crawford and Barbara Stanwyck to the cast of the smash-hit series "Dynasty." We met during the casting of the pilot for another hit series, "Charlie's Angels," for which he designed throughout its five-year run. Nolan has become a friend, as well as a trusted co-worker who has dressed me for several films and personal appearances since.

JS: I realized as we worked together on "Charlie's Angels" that one of the difficulties in designing clothes for a series is keeping those clothes contemporary without letting them get too dated. Is that a good rule of thumb for any woman to follow in building her wardrobe?

NM: Absolutely. I always advise women to avoid buying clothes that are so "of the moment," so trendy that someone's bound to comment the next season: "Oh, I loved that look!" with the emphasis on the past tense. Let's face it, clothes are expensive and almost no woman has a truly unlimited budget. Accessories are where you can indulge your passion for the "latest" without breaking the bank.

Let me give you an example. Several seasons ago, star motifs and patterns were very hot. The smart woman went out and bought a star-printed scarf or a star-shaped rhinestone pin instead of plunking down hundreds of dollars on a star-patterned silk dress that would now be at the back of her closet because it's too identifiable as "old."

JS: I know you believe in working out a wardrobe based on a few key colors. How does a woman decide which are her colors? Does she consider her hair color, skin tone or just go with her favorites?

NM: The answer is, all of the above. But of primary importance, I think, is that she feels comfortable in the color. No matter how good someone else thinks you look in green, if you don't like green . . .

Second, the complexion determines good color ranges and depths. A sallow-skinned person wants to avoid yellow and yellow-greens at all costs. A lady with a lot of red in her face would probably stay away from reds, fuchsias, red-purples. A very white, pale complexion usually rules out wearing white because it washes the person out. But

*Reflecting my own taste for body-skimming evening gowns, this dress was designed by Nolan Miller for my role in **The Users**.*

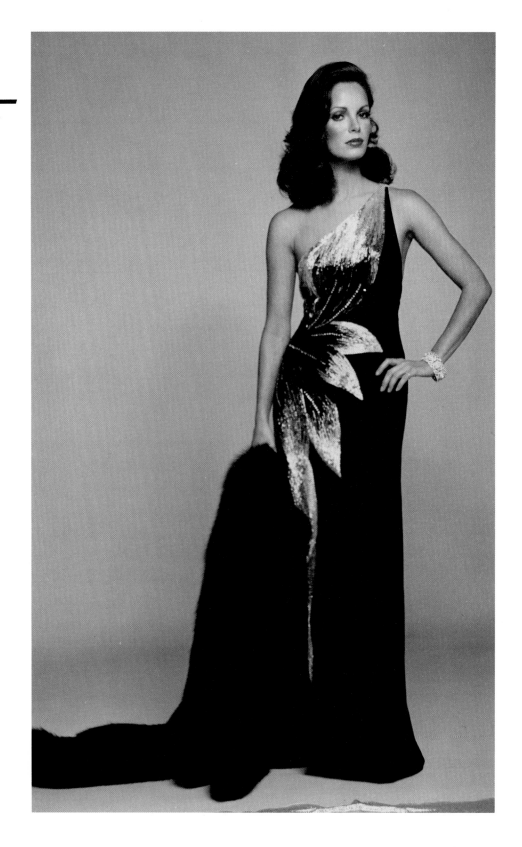

I do not believe in those old rules about blondes' wearing only pale pink, blue and white. Or redheads' wearing only greens.

JS: Given that nobody's perfect, how should a woman approach figure faults?

NM: Be honest about them. I mean it. She has to look in the mirror and see that her hips are too broad, or whatever. And she mustn't forget to check the back view. A critical analysis of how you look "leaving the scene" is important, too.

JS: What sorts of styles are right if your hips are big?

NM: Well, you'd certainly not want to squeeze those hips into too-tight jeans or wrap them with a red sash, just because that's the current fashion. I'd advise clothes that play up the upper torso: interesting necklines and off-the-shoulder dresses, for example.

JS: What if you're big-bosomed?

NM: A lot of women think they can overcome a too-ample bust by wearing something that's very tight across the chest. Tight doesn't make you look smaller; it just makes you look like you're about to burst out or fall out of your clothes. But covered-up, high-necked styles are often good, and wearing all one color on top helps minimize a big bust. Needless to say, ruffles and empire waistlines are out of the question.

JS: What about petite women? Are they left out when it comes to high fashion?

NM: Not at all. They just have to be a bit more subtle, and usually look best if they aren't wearing a lot of different colors or a big, busy print. A neutral shoe also helps because it lengthens the leg/foot line, and hems should be kept around the knee. Forget show-stopping effects like picture hats and fox, or any long-haired, fur.

JS: What's a woman to do if she's short-waisted?

NM: I wouldn't advise a severely defined waist—for instance, a wide, wide belt. And if she's a little top-heavy, a white blouse and black skirt, that is, light on top, dark on the bottom, is the opposite of the right approach. Ideally, she should wear outfits in two tones of the same color.

JS: Very tall women must be the luckiest of all, since clothes seem to be designed with five-foot-ten-inch models in mind.

NM: It's true that taller women can carry off long-haired furs, shoulder-padded looks and big-scale patterns. What they have to watch is vertical stripes and too-long skirts that can really "stretch them out" too much.

JS: They say you can't be too thin. But surely ultrathin women have to make some adjustments in choosing silhouettes that are most flattering?

NM: I believe a woman *can* be too thin, and there's nothing I find less attractive, less sexy than a lot of bareness on these women. To see bony shoulders and stringy necks sticking out of strapless or one-shoulder gowns is awful, I think. I would advise these women to keep covered up. Or, if they want to be sexy, reveal a smooth back.

Actually, to me, fabric is the thing that makes a dress or an outfit sexy. It's not the obvious bareness. What could be lovelier, more appealing than a fluid, body-clinging silk jersey or satin-back crepe?

JS: Nearly every woman in America has been ten pounds overweight at some point. Can you dress "thinner"?

NM: There are some obvious things you can do to minimize a little extra weight, but I always say, "There's no substitute for a good diet!" I'm constantly being asked by producers to dress an actor or an

Soft jerseys and knits make for fresh-looking, comfortable clothes that can take you from a business meeting to an alfresco lunch.

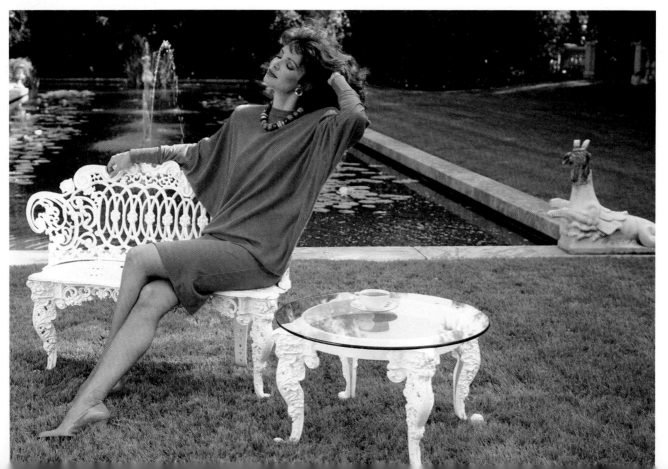

actress so he or she looks slimmer. After a certain point—about ten pounds—there's nothing I can do.

When I see that one of the actresses I know well is putting on weight, I simply, subtly let the word "matronly" slip into our conversation, and she always gets the hint. It's as if a gong goes off.

JS: You know I like to wear things that my husband, Tony, likes. But whom should a woman look to for advice on choosing her clothes? Her girlfriends? Salespeople?

NM: I believe a woman should first of all please herself, but there's nothing wrong with pleasing the man in her life, either. I know so many women who've bought things that are gathering dust now because the husband or boyfriend hates it. Taking the advice of girlfriends or salespeople is risky because they're bound to impose their own tastes, which often has nothing to do with what's suitable and flattering for you.

JS: Are there some items that you think are inappropriate for a woman of "a certain age"?

NM: I do, indeed. My pet peeve of all time is seeing a fifty-year-old woman with long, Alice in Wonderland hair streaming down her back. And no matter what her figure, I think an older woman should skip the ultrashort skirts, tight jeans and, as I've said, bare, bare dresses.

JS: I know you're a firm believer in the impact accessories can make. Any general principles that apply here?

NM: Well, I already mentioned the point about neutral shoes. I don't believe in gimmicky or brightly colored shoes that call attention to themselves. That's the last place you want people to look when they're observing you.

I realize that the day won't come again when a woman would rather go outside without her shoes on than appear without a hat, but I still believe hats can be wonderful additions to a look. I especially like little cocktail hats with veils; men love their mysterious flirtatiousness. But hats are really for women with today's shorter hairstyles.

Handbags are sort of like shoes: subtly colored—not meant to *match* an outfit—and unobtrusive ones are best.

I'm a big fan of costume jewelry, carefully chosen and worn. I have

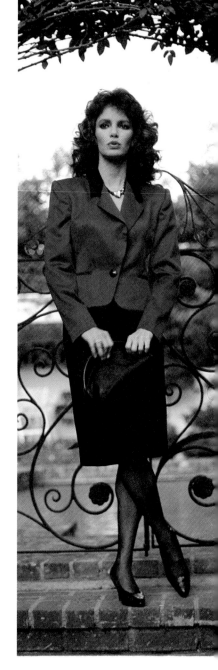

Just-right proportions and a few well-chosen accessories create a smart daytime look.

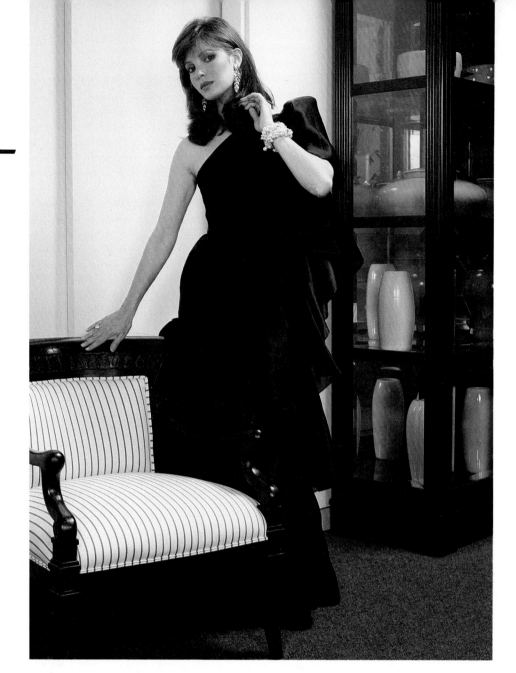

one very personal exception, though. I have never liked long, dangling earrings. But then, that's just my taste.

JS: What are the biggest problems women have with getting their "look" together?

NM: There are two things that I'd mention. First, we've had several years now when young women have worn jeans and sweaters. They don't spend time as teenagers and young women trying on and experimenting with their mothers' "real" clothes. In fact, for a while, I guess the mothers themselves didn't have much beyond jeans and tops.

I think that's changing now, though, and as fashion continues to present dressed-up options—suits, dresses, long skirts, etc.—again, I hope young women will grow up with more experience about clothes. You'd be surprised at the number of actresses in their twenties who have no idea how to wear an evening dress or high heels!

My point is that it takes time to learn what sorts of clothes look best on you, to find your niche. I hope young girls are getting that "training" these days, as they used to.

The second thing I notice is that women invariably make a mistake when they don't plan ahead, when they want to look great for an occasion that's important to them. Rushing out and buying a dress to wear to a big dinner the same night is, nine times out of ten, a disaster.

And it's important to take a little time, *before* your husband is standing in the front hall shouting that you're late, to get the right stockings, the right belt, the right things together. I'm not talking about being a slave to your look, just making the most of your efforts to dress well and be attractive.

JS: You travel and work a lot in Europe. How would you define American style versus European?

NM: For the most part, I think Europeans have a subtler approach to dressing. We Americans are more into "statement" clothes, and that makes a great deal of sense since this is a country of strong individualism. One example is that we wear many more bright colors, especially during the day. To me, American style means vitality and variety. There's an extraordinary range of choices for women today; it's just that slightly tricky question of choosing well—for you!

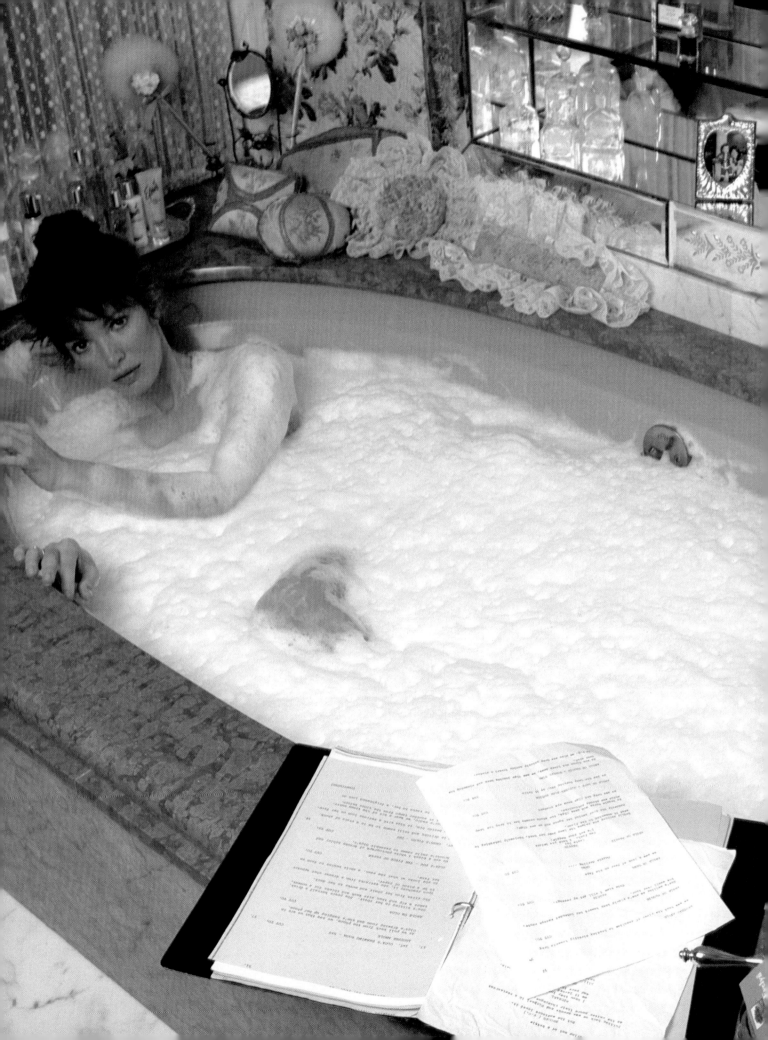

CHAPTER 11

Bath: The Great Escape

As long as I can remember, I've loved baths. When I was a child, my mother never had to cajole me into the tub, and when I was a teenager, I think she often found me pretty tough to extract. I used to lie in the bath until I was positively prune-y! There is nothing more relaxing, more satisfying after a busy day than a hot bath, especially in winter. And I do mean *really* hot!

I know the practically scalding water I prefer can be scalding to skin, and some people claim that a hot bath makes you sleepy. But not for me. The experience goes way beyond clean—a rather nice feeling in itself—to giving me a sense of exuberance.

I'm so lucky that in our home I've been able to create my dream bathroom. It's full of frilly, feminine things, and Tony can't complain because he's got his own, strictly masculine bathroom, all in forest green tones and verdigris marble, on the other side of the bedroom.

Mine is a large rectangular room, papered in giant, old-fashioned cabbage roses, with lots of pink and white marble detailing. The Jacuzzi tub is rimmed in delicately beveled rose marble, and has a

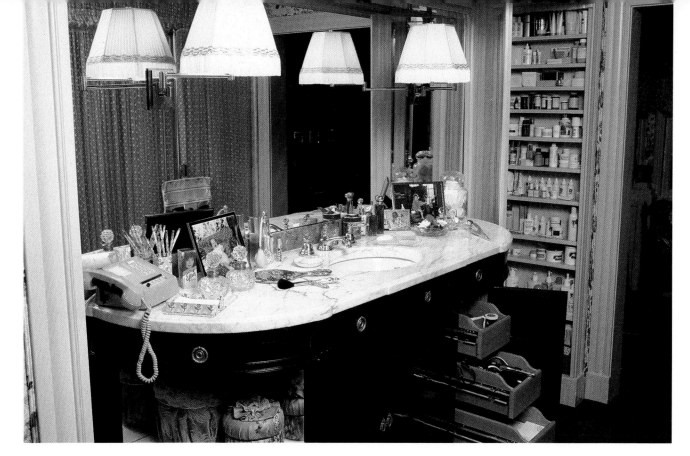

There's fierce organization behind what appears to be my purely decorative bathroom.

mirrored shadow box over it, where I display all my perfume bottles and Battersea boxes. There are lace pillows, baskets of pretty soaps and potpourri, and often, vases of fresh-cut flowers all around the tub.

The pièce de résistance, I think, is my sink, hand-painted with a flowers-and-ribbons design, set into an antique mahogany sideboard-like piece. I've had the inside of this cabinet fitted with ultramodern sliding drawers custom-designed to hold all the beauty basics: one drawer for makeup, one for hair combs and ribbons, one each to hold a hand-held hair dryer, a hood-type dryer, and my heat lamps—for when I want to leave my hair natural. The most clever part is that all the electrical connections are out of sight, in back, and I never have to fiddle with plugging anything in. The dryers are always ready to go. I love having everything organized, and best of all, hidden away when I'm not using it.

The room is large enough to include a full steam shower and, at the other end, in a little windowed niche, my antique writing table and a sofa. As you can see, my bath really is a great escape for me, a place of total peace and privacy, where I can indulge my hopelessly romantic attitudes. Scattered as it is with family photos and precious mementos, it's my ultrafeminine fantasy world. I suppose it sounds

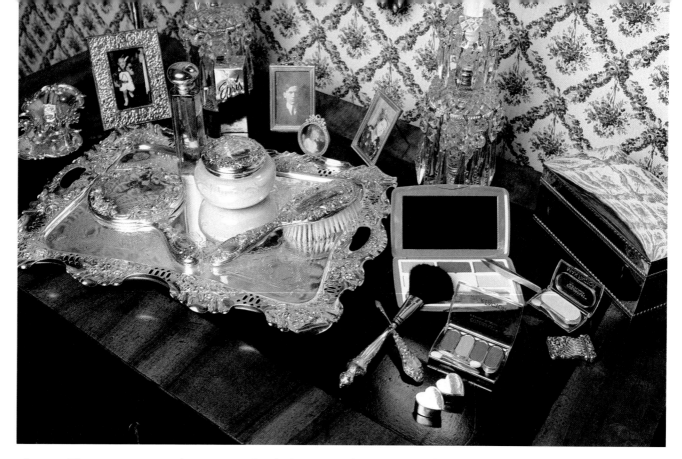

almost like a stage set, but I simply feel so good surrounded by so many pretty things.

Beloved photos and personal mementos make my bathroom a private, personal sanctuary.

CREATE YOUR OWN SENSUAL SPA

Even if you aren't able to claim a whole bathroom for yourself, there's so much you can do to make the daily bathing ritual a deeply soothing, relaxing experience.

First of all, no one ever decreed that you have to bathe in full-wattage lighting: dim the lights or even just bathe by candlelight. It's a great way to set the mood for a tension-reducing soak. Music, a radio or tape recorder, is a good idea. And why not scent the entire scene? I've found a vanilla-based room spray that's become an addiction.

Pampering yourself does take a little beforehand preparation. Have a favorite, warm, terry robe ready, as well as a fresh towel and scented soap; a liquid called Bain Crème Vanille is my first choice. Skin-conditioning bubbling gels or lightly scented oils, especially if you're a hot-water enthusiast like me, are lovely options, too.

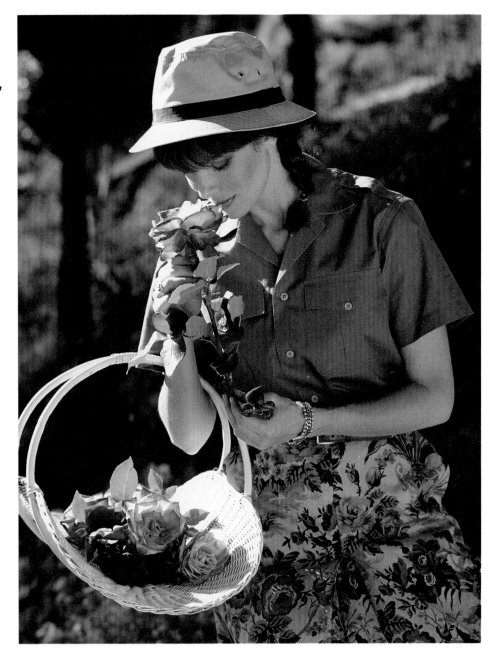

The condition of the water itself is important. As I've learned only too well from travels across this country and around the world, hard water can wreak havoc with your skin and hair. How many times have I been discouraged with the lack of shine in my just-washed hair when in England, for example? Well, here in our own home, as I've told you, we've found the answer in a water-softening unit that services the whole house. We simply have to feed it rock salt about once

EASY POTPOURRI

Making your own potpourri—as a room scenter displayed in decorated baskets, a china bowl, or teacup or to enclose in little cheesecloth, drawstring bags for steeping—isn't really difficult at all.

You simply pick fresh ingredients for color and scent. I love combinations that include lavender buds, rose petals, the leaves of an orange tree, mint or lemon verbena with cinnamon or vanilla beans for their fragrance and dried pansies and, maybe, marigolds for color. You can use crumbled flowers and leaves, or whole buds. The key is to allow every ingredient to dry out completely, and then blend them all together with a fixative, like orris root or musk oil.

Tuck your mixture away in a tightly sealed container for up to seven weeks, and the whole thing will sort of mulch into a wonderful, *custom* potpourri. (As a matter of fact, it's good to note the specific ingredients and their relative amounts, to have a permanent record of your favorite potpourri experiment.)

---

a month. I'm so adamant on this point that I'd rather have to rinse more often to get the soap off in soft water, than deal with the harshness of hard.

Since I have a quite successful herb and flower garden on the property, I'm also able to indulge every once in a while, when I have the time, in wonderful natural baths. As well as drying flower petals and herbs for potpourri, to scent the room, you can create fragrant liquid "sachets" to bathe in. All you have to do is dry about a cupful of mixed blossom petals and then steep them in boiling water, a cup-and-a-half or two, like tea. After about fifteen minutes, pour the mixture into the just-run bathwater.

Even simpler than that is tossing a few teaspoons of mixed, dried herbs directly into the tub: sage, rosemary, mint and thyme are all good choices. The only caveat here is to be careful when your bathwater is draining, to be sure it doesn't clog.

If yours has been an active, muscle-wrenching day, you might resort to the soothing powers of plain, old-fashioned baking soda. (I have to credit Gaston and his occasional bouts of diaper rash for this discovery.) This back-of-the-pantry staple is a super inflammation-reducer for grown-up sunburns, too.

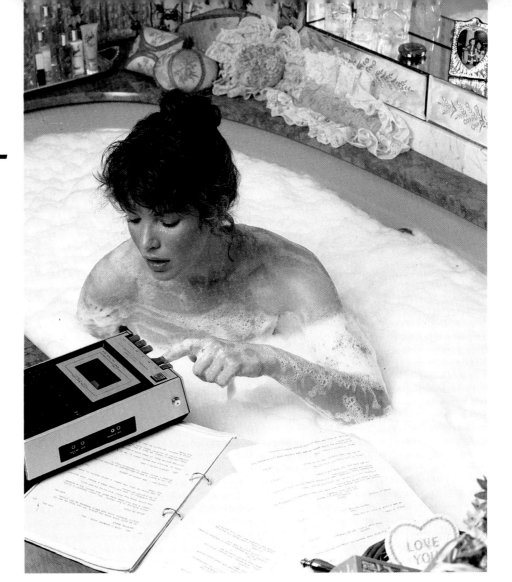

I often settle into the tub with a script and my tape recorder at hand. The tapes contain my dialogue sessions with my coach, so I can learn my lines almost subliminally, hearing myself say them over and over again as I bathe. But the bath is also a super time to delve into a compelling Gothic romance novel or simply to enjoy music you love. (No electrical appliances too near the tub, of course.)

Instead of the Jacuzzi or any other water-jet system, you can achieve muscle-soothing benefits with a semirough loofah massage mitt, or one of those rubber-nippled massagers, available in drugstores. Massage, coupled with the pleasure of being submerged in warm water, feels great!

Everything changes when Gaston joins me for a bath. Then it's more like a swimming pool. Lots of boats and toys and splashing and giggling. And he certainly doesn't go for the water temperature I prefer. But it's a very close time, and something I wouldn't miss for

JACLYN SMITH'S BATHTIME-RETREAT SURVIVAL KIT

If a bathroom cluttered with tub toys and your man's shaving gear doesn't immediately inspire you to thoughts of an indulgent spa, I suggest you develop a "survival kit." By that I mean a big wicker basket—you could paint it yourself, and a lid might discourage prying and raiding—stocked with your bath-retreat goodies so it's ready whenever you are. Here, a checklist:

1 large basket
1 fresh bath towel or bath sheet
1 fresh, smaller towel
1 facecloth or natural sponge
1 backbrush or loofah mitt
1 bath pillow
fragrant soaps
potpourri or liquid sachet
bubble bath
scented candles
favorite tapes and a cassette player
hair ribbons or a pretty shower cap
body lotion
dusting powder

the world, even if it means bathing all over again later, after he's gone to bed.

When I finally, always reluctantly, drag myself out of the tub, I dry off with a towel and smooth on lots of quick-penetrating body lotion, neck to toes, before slipping into a cozy robe or the lingerie I stash in fabric-covered boxes, right there in the bathroom. If I'm going to bed, I often like to finish with scented dusting powder, for a subtler-than-perfume, allover fragrance.

SHOWER POWER

You've surely got the picture: I love nothing more than a long, languorous bath. But when I'm filming, which often means rising before the sun, I opt for the steam shower in the morning.

It's not an experience totally lacking in pleasure, though. For instance, I sometimes tie a little drawstring sack of herbal potpourri so that the water runs through it, scenting the environment and adding an extra invigorating element. I also take advantage of the steam's penetration effect to have a mini-deep-cleansing facial while I shower: I apply a rich cream, like Albolene, and leave it on my face throughout the shower.

Even without a professional steam shower, you can enjoy steam-cleaning by tenting your head under a towel, as you expose your face to the steam from a bowl of steaming water. Either way, you're left with glowing, soft, clean skin.

I also wash and condition my hair every morning in the shower, rinsing with first lukewarm, then ice-cold water. Believe me, that'll wake you up!

Take your loofah mitt or massager into the shower with you. Or, what about getting one of those pulsating shower-head attachments so widely available now? They're all great ways to loosen up sleep-stiff muscles and make you ready to meet the day!

DOUBLE YOUR PLEASURE

Bathtime is the perfect opportunity to treat yourself to a facial mask and save precious time by accomplishing two things at once. Since Tony's vegetable garden yields such delicious, and handy, specimens, I often get a ripe avocado from it, for my own purposes. One table-spoon of avocado flesh, mashed up with two tablespoons of honey and a whole egg is one of the nicest things you'll *ever* do for your face. I admit this mask is a touch tricky to wash off, but it's well worth the minimum extra effort because of its natural, skin-enriching qualities.

If you're even more of a purist, you can take the plain, ripe avocado meat, smash it up as you warm it over a double boiler, then apply it to your face just like that. After fifteen to twenty minutes, rinse with warm, then cool water.

Needless to say, any mask, homemade or not, makes sense when you're in the private world of your bath. Their effects are many and marvelous—cleansing, pore-tightening, skin-smoothing—but you're not very pretty to look at when you're wearing them.

If tired-looking and -feeling eyes are your complaint, just lean back and relax in the tub with two fresh, crisp cucumber slices—yes,

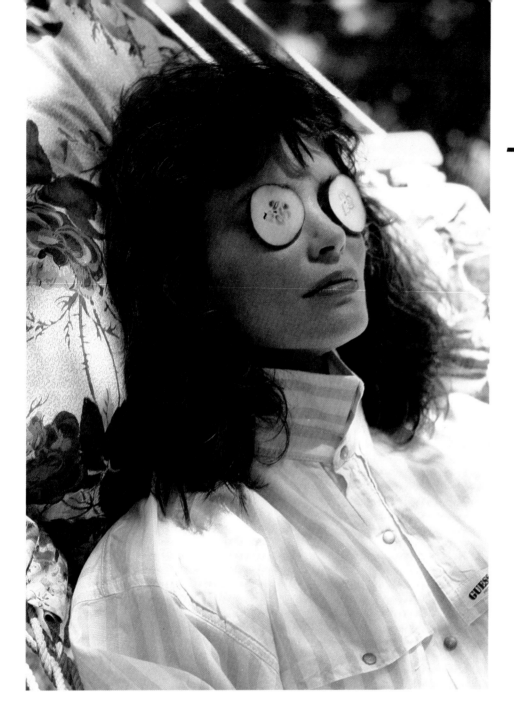

*The backyard vegetable
garden provides the freshest
natural eye soothers.*

Tony's garden again—on your eyelids. Slightly damp tea bags or
those commercial ice-pack eye masks (the ones that make you look
like a feminine version of the Lone Ranger, in pale aqua) work just as
well to reduce any puffiness and redness. But I love the idea of the
cucumber's straight-from-nature magic powers.

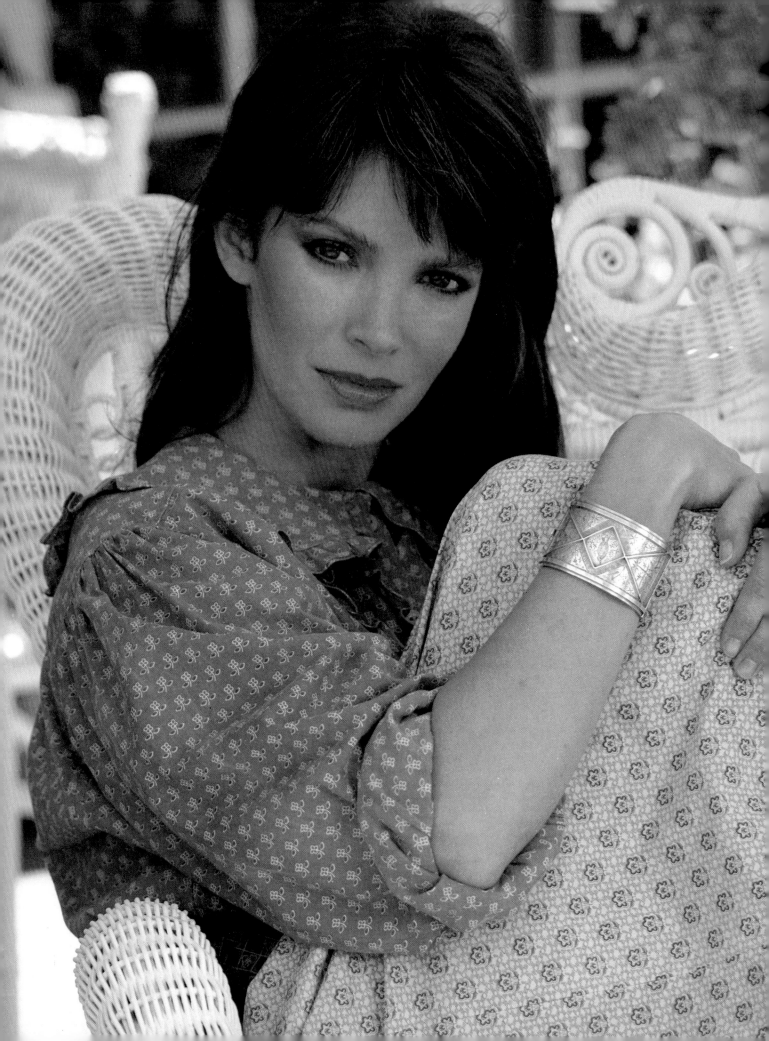

Epilogue

When I began this project, I was a bit hesitant. I mean, I am not the ultimate beauty expert, and the notion of writing a whole book on the American look seemed somehow, well, self-centered. As it has turned out, I've enjoyed the process tremendously because I've learned as much as you have about finding one's own distinct style, one's way, one's look.

Working on this book has only reconfirmed my conviction that liking yourself—the real you—is the key to truly feminine, American beauty. This book's purpose is far from being a manual on becoming a Jaclyn Smith clone. In fact, the goal is the opposite. While learning a lot of useful information about getting a great body, having healthy, shining hair, glowing skin and pretty makeup, I think we've established a single, overriding theme: when we talk about you becoming beautiful, the most significant word in the sentence is "you." Any experiments, any new techniques in self-improvement, must yield an individualized, prettier, more self-confident you, otherwise it's really not worth the effort.

If I've nudged you into taking better care of yourself, that's great. If I've inspired you to try new looks, new ideas, so much the better. But the heart of my message is this: simply be the best *you* can. I firmly believe there can be no beauty without happiness, and no happiness without self-discovery *and* self-acceptance.

With love,

PHOTO CREDITS

All of the photographs in this book were taken by Charles William Bush, with the exception of those listed below, which are used by permission and which the author gratefully acknowledges.

American Broadcasting Company: pp. 34, 36, 172
Canon Films, Ltd.: p. 51
Bob Greene/Columbia Broadcasting System: p. 40
Health and Tennis Corporation of America: p. 145
© John Breck & Co., Courtesy American Cyanamid Company/Shulton, Inc. U.S.A.: p. 33
Harris Johnston: p. 32
Klaus Lukas/Max Factor: p. 41
National Broadcasting Company: p. 54
Barrie Payne/Canon Films, Ltd.: p. 19
Dr. and Mrs. Smith: pp. 12, 32
Charles Varon: pp. 13, 14
Raul Vega: pp. 152, 154
Alana Voeller: p. 47
© Wella Balsam: p. 33